High-Yield Pharmacology

High-Yield Pharmacology

Daryl Christ, Ph.D.

Associate Professor of Pharmacology

South Bend Center for Medical Education

Indiana University School of Medicine

Notre Dame, Indiana

 LIPPINCOTT WILLIAMS & WILKINS

A **Wolters Kluwer** Company

Philadelphia · Baltimore · New York · London
Buenos Aires · Hong Kong · Sydney · Tokyo

Editor: Elizabeth A. Nieginski
Development Editors: Rosanne Hallowell, Emilie Linkins
Marketing Manager: Jennifer Conrad
Managing Editor: Karla M. Schroeder

351 West Camden Street
Baltimore, Maryland 21201-2436 USA

530 Walnut Street
Philadelphia, Pennsylvania 19106-3621

The publisher is not responsible (as a matter of product liability, negligence or other-
wise) for any injury resulting from any material contained herein. This publication contains information relating to general principles of medical care which should not be
construed as specific instructions for individual patients. Manufacturers' product information and package inserts should be reviewed for current information, including contraindications, dosages and precautions.

Printed in the United States of America

Library of Congress Cataloging-in-Publication Data

Christ, Daryl
    High-yield pharmacology / Daryl Christ.
        p.   cm. — (High-yield series)
    Based on the author's 1988 self-published work: Pharmacology in a nutshell.
    ISBN 0-683-30713-4
    1. Pharmacology—Outlines, syllabi, etc.   I. Title.   II.   Series
    [DNLM: 1. Pharmacology outlines.   QV 18.2 C554h 1999]
    RM301.14.C48   1999
    615'.1—dc21
    DNLM/DLC   98-52915
    for Library of Congress   CIP

*The publishers have made every effort to trace the copyright holders for borrowed material. If
they have inadvertently overlooked any, they will be pleased to make the necessary arrange-
ments at the first opportunity.*

To purchase additional copies of this book, call our customer service department at
(800) 638-3030 or fax orders to **(301) 824-7390.** International customers should call
(301) 714-2324.

00 01 02 03
3 4 5 6 7 8 9 10

Contents

Preface

First, the name is pronounced Christ, as in Christ-ian, Christ-mas, or Christ-opher. As the son of farmers, Esther and George Christ, I learned at an early age to reduce life to a few simple principles. In my 30 years of teaching pharmacology, the benefits of using such an approach to prepare students for the United States Medical Licensing Examination (USMLE) have become obvious.

In 1988, the first (self-published) edition of my concise review guide *Pharmacology in a Nutshell* was written and distributed to the Indiana University medical students at the South Bend Center for Medical Education. Since then it has been adopted by each statewide Indiana University medical class, and in recent years the classes have taken over the task of coping, binding, and distributing the *Pharmacology in a Nutshell* to all the Indiana University sophomore medical students. Since 1991, I have also been presenting a 7-hour review of pharmacology, given in 1 day, to each statewide Indiana University sophomore medical class. This is held about 2 weeks before the USMLE Step 1, and more than half of the students attend this session. The students have frequently commented that most of the material needed for the examination was covered in *Pharmacology in a Nutshell*.

High-Yield Pharmacology is based on *Pharmacology in a Nutshell*. It contains essentially the same material, but in the outline format of the High-Yield series. The underlying premise for both reviews is that a good grasp of the major concepts of pharmacology is better than a poor grasp of all the concepts of pharmacology. In this regard, it is best to study the drugs as classes, rather than as individual drugs. Begin by studying the prototype drug for each class, and then expand on this by studying the other drugs in the class that have unique differences from the prototype. Only generic names are used on the examination. However, in this book the trade name, or an example of one trade name for that generic drug, have been provided for informational purposes. These trade names are indicated in parentheses and italic type and are placed directly after the corresponding generic name. No dosages and very few chemical structures need to be remembered for the USMLE Step 1. Memorization of long lists of mundane side effects, detailed kinetic properties, and detailed mechanisms of action is usually not required. Instead, the most important or the unique properties of the drugs should be studied. Many pharmacological principles evolved from the autonomic drugs, so a thorough understanding of this class of drugs is essential.

My background in teaching medical pharmacology began at the University of Arkansas College of Medicine in 1970. I left Arkansas in 1983 to take a position on the faculty of the Indiana University School of Medicine, where I still teach. During that time, I have received a Pre-Clinical Science Golden Apple Award (1981), a Runner-Up Pre-Clinical Science Golden Apple Award (1983), an Outstanding Professor in Basic Sciences Teaching Award (1993) and a Teaching Excellence Recognition Award (1998).

The statewide program at Indiana University is a truly unique medical education program, in which half of each freshman and sophomore medical class attends at Indianapolis and the other half of the class is divided among 8 university campuses for their basic science courses. The small Center for Medical Education provides me with an opportunity to teach the complete pharmacology course by myself to a group of 14–16 sophomore medical students. This format allows for consistent coverage of all the material in an organized fashion.

This review book, *High Yield Pharmacology*, in a format proven to be effective for medical students studying for USMLE Step 1, similarly provides consistent, concise, and comprehensive coverage.

Daryl Christ

Acknowledgments

The author would like to acknowledge some of the people who have had a major impact on his life. First and foremost are his wife Bonnie and his son Alan, who, as an artist and an architect, respectively, always remind him that life is more than just science. The author would also like to acknowledge his parents, Esther and George Christ, and older brothers, Don and Duane Christ, who were so important during his formative and later years. Others will recognize their initials, including friends from Lakota High School in Iowa (DWC), Wartburg College (DAH and CDK), University of Iowa (ARB), and Loyola University in Chicago (JWG, TJS, JPG, PSG, RSJ, and NJD).

It has also been the author's good fortune to work with some excellent pharmacologists and educators, including Leslie C. Blaber, Alexander G. Karczmar, and Syogoro Nishi at Loyola University in Chicago; Werner E. Flacke and Donald E. McMillan at the University of Arkansas; Henry R. Besch, Jr., Thomas A. Troeger, and John F. O'Malley at Indiana University; and Howard J. Saz at the University of Notre Dame.

The author especially wishes to acknowledge the efforts of Ann Selzer, M.D., Internal Medicine, who reviewed the initial draft for this book and provided thoughtful comments.

1

General Principles

I. ABSORPTION AND DISTRIBUTION OF DRUGS

A. **Pharmacokinetics** is the study of the movement of drugs into and out of the body, including **uptake, distribution, biotransformation,** and **elimination.**

B. The movement of drugs across cell membranes usually occurs by **diffusion.**

C. The rate of diffusion is high if:

1. **The unionized form of a drug has a high lipid solubility.**
   a. The lipid solubility is related to the oil-water partition coefficient.
   b. Cell membranes are basically lipoidal in nature, and only lipid soluble substances will diffuse through them.

2. **A large proportion of the drug is present in the unionized form.**
   a. **Only the unionized form can cross cell membranes,** because the ionized form will have a very low solubility in lipids.
   b. The equilibrium between the ionized (A^-) and unionized (HA) forms of a weak acid is:

$$HA \rightleftharpoons H^+ + A^-$$

   c. The proportion of unionized drug will depend on the pH and can be determined with the Henderson-Hasselbach equation.
   d. For a drug that is a weak acid, the equation is:

$$pK_a = pH + \log \frac{[\text{unionized}]}{[\text{ionized}]}$$

   e. Weak bases also dissociate, and the equilibrium for a weak base is:

$$B + H^+ \rightleftharpoons BH^+$$

   f. The Henderson-Hasselbach relationship for a weak base is:

$$pK_a = pH + \log \frac{[\text{ionized}]}{[\text{unionized}]}$$

   g. The ratio of unionized to ionized drug concentrations for a weak base is the inverse of the ratio for a weak acid.

   h. When the pH equals the pK_a, 50% of a drug will be ionized and 50% will be unionized.

    i. The biggest changes in the amounts of ionized and unionized drug occur with pH changes near the pK_a.

   3. The membrane is thin.

   4. The membrane is porous. Porosity is especially important for water-soluble drugs.

   5. The surface area of the membrane is large.

   6. The difference in concentrations on the two sides of the membrane is large.

   7. The diffusion constant, based on molecular size, molecular shape, and temperature, is large.

D. At the **low pH** in the stomach:

   1. Weak acids are well absorbed because most of the drug is unionized.

   2. Weak bases are poorly absorbed because most of the drug is ionized.

E. Ion trapping occurs with weak acids and weak bases if there is a difference in pH on the two sides of a membrane.

   1. The ionized form of the drug will be trapped on one side.

     a. The ionized form of a **weak base** will be trapped on the side with the **lower pH.**

     b. The ionized form of a **weak acid** will be trapped on the side with the **higher pH.**

   2. Figure 1–1 illustrates ion trapping for a weak acid with a pK_a of 6.4. At equilibrium, the unionized concentrations on either side of the membrane will be equal, but 91% of the drug will be in the compartment at pH 7.4.

F. Strong bases and **strong acids** are **totally dissociated** or ionized in solution; thus, they are **poorly absorbed at any pH.** Quaternary ammonium compounds are completely ionized at physiological pHs and therefore are also poorly absorbed.

G. Many routes of drug administration can be used.

   1. The **oral route** (PO) is usually preferred.

     a. Advantages include:

       (1) Convenience

Figure 1-1.   Ion trapping of a weak acid (pK_a 6.4) on the side of the cell membrane with the higher pH. The numbers in parentheses represent the relative concentrations of each form of the weak acid under steady state conditions.

        (2) A **large surface area** for absorption

        (3) Less abrupt changes of serum drug concentrations than with parenteral administration

    b. **A major disadvantage is first pass metabolism** by the liver.

        (1) All the blood flow from the intestinal tract goes initially to the liver through the portal vein; therefore, the **drug may be metabolized before being distributed** to the other tissues in the body.

        (2) First pass metabolism of a drug can be **avoided by sublingual administration** and partially avoided by rectal administration.

  2. The **parenteral routes** of administration are technically more difficult and usually must be performed by a health care professional.

    a. **Advantages** include:

        (1) A faster onset (usually)

        (2) More reliable absorption

        (3) No first pass metabolism

    b. **Disadvantages** include:

        (1) More difficult administration

        (2) Pain or necrosis at the site of injection

        (3) Possibility of **infection**

        (4) Toxicity from a bolus intravenous (IV) injection

        (5) Necessity of dissolving the drug if given intravenously

H. The **initial distribution** of a drug to the tissues is determined by the **relative blood flows** to the tissues. Sites with high blood flows will initially receive more of the drug.

I. The final distribution, also called the **apparent volume of distribution (V_d),** will be affected by:

  1. **The lipid solubility** of a drug, which, if high, will result in good penetration into cells.

  2. **Plasma protein binding and tissue binding**

    a. **Plasma protein binding, especially to albumin,** will reduce the V_d.

    b. **Tissue binding** will increase the V_d.

    c. Both types of binding act as **reservoirs** for the drug, as only the unbound drug can activate pharmacological receptors. Thus binding will:

        (1) Slow the onset of drug action

        (2) Prolong the duration of drug action, if the drug is eliminated by glomerular filtration in the kidney

II. METABOLISM OF DRUGS

  A. The **liver** is the **primary site of drug metabolism.**

  B. Metabolism can change a drug in several ways.

    1. The **polarity is usually increased,** enhancing the water solubility and renal excretion of the drug metabolite.

    2. The **activity of the drug is reduced. Exceptions** are the **prodrugs,** which are drugs that are inactive in the form administered but are metabolized to their active forms.

    3. Drug metabolites usually have **smaller V_d.**

  C. **Phase 1** metabolic reactions lead to the **degradation** of the drug.

    1. **Oxidation by mixed function oxidases (MFO)** [also known as cytochrome P450s, microsomal enzymes, mono-oxygenases] **occurs** in the **smooth endoplasmic reticulum (ER).**

   a. Nicotinamide adenine dinucleotide phosphate (NADPH), **cytochrome P450 reductase,** and elemental oxygen (O_2) are required.

   b. Many reactions can be produced, including:

     (1) Hydroxylation
     (2) Dealkylation
     (3) Deamination
     (4) Sulfoxidation
     (5) Oxidation

   c. Highly lipid soluble drugs are more readily metabolized by MFOs.

  2. Reductive reactions can occur in the ER or the cytosol.

  3. Hydrolytic reactions do not occur in the ER.

D. Phase 2 metabolic reactions are **conjugative** (synthetic).

  1. Glucuronidation occurs in the **ER.** Glucose is used to form uridine diphosphate glucuronic acid (UDPGA) which then transfers a glucuronide to the drug in the presence of glucuronyl transferase.

  2. Other substances can also be conjugated (by transferases) to drugs, thereby reducing the drug activity, including:

   a. Sulfate
   b. Acetyl
   c. Methyl
   d. Glutathione
   e. Amino acids, especially glycine

E. Many drug **interactions** result from changes in MFO activity in the liver.

  1. Induction of MFOs results from increased levels of MFOs in the ER.

   a. The onset of induction is **slow** (days) and the duration is **long** (taking a week or more for recovery).

   b. Many drugs that are metabolized by the MFOs induce the MFOs, including

     (1) Barbiturates, phenytoin, rifampin, warfarin
     (2) Alcohol
     (3) Cigarette smoke

   c. This induction hastens the metabolism of the inducing drug and many other drugs.

  2. Enzyme inhibition occurs if there is **competition** between drugs (e.g., cimetidine), for the MFO.

III. EXCRETION OF DRUGS AND DRUG METABOLITES

A. The **kidney** is the primary organ that excretes drugs and drug metabolites.

  1. If the drug is excreted in the unmetabolized form, the kidney also decreases the pharmacological activity.

  2. Polar drugs and **polar drug metabolites** are readily eliminated by the kidney.

B. Filtration of the unbound molecule accounts for the excretion of most drugs.

  1. Drug bound by plasma proteins will not be filtered by the glomerulus.

  2. Hydrophilic or lipophobic substances are most **efficiently eliminated** by the kidney, because they are not readily reabsorbed across the nephron tubule after they are filtered.

   3. If a drug is a **weak base,** administration of ammonium chloride will **acidify the urine** and increase the amount of the base that is in the ionized form.
      a. The excretion of the weak base will be increased.
      b. This will be most effective if the pK_a of the drug is near the physiological pH.

C. **Active transport** of a few drugs occurs in the **proximal tubule.**

   1. It usually involves **secretion of strong acids or strong bases.**

   2. **Characteristics** of active transport are:
      a. **Competition** between substrates for the carrier
      b. **Saturation** of the carrier
      c. **Being unaffected by plasma protein binding**

   3. **Active reabsorption** can also occur.

   4. A few substances are both actively secreted and actively reabsorbed (e.g., uric acid, aspirin).

D. **Biliary excretion** occurs in the liver.

   1. **Large polar compounds,** often conjugated metabolites, are actively excreted into the bile.

   2. **Enterohepatic cycling** occurs with a few drugs that are eliminated in the bile, re-absorbed from the intestine, returned to the liver and again eliminated in the bile.
      a. **Glucuronidase** in the intestine can cleave off the glucuronide, so the free drug can be reabsorbed (Figure 1–2).
      b. **Digitoxin,** a cardiac glycoside, undergoes enterohepatic cycling.
      c. This **may increase the half-life** of the drug.

IV. CLINICAL PHARMACOKINETICS

A. Clinical pharmacokinetics, which involves the **mathematical description** of the **processes of drug absorption, distribution, metabolism,** and **elimination,** is useful to predict the serum drug concentrations under various conditions.

B. **Absorption of a drug is usually fast,** as compared to the elimination; thus, it is often ignored in kinetic calculations.

C. **Elimination** usually follows the principles of **first-order kinetics,** which means that a constant fraction of the drug is eliminated per unit of time (K_e).

D. Several **equations** are useful.

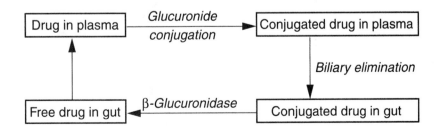

Figure 1-2.   Enterohepatic cycling of a conjugated drug.

1. Bioavailability (F) equation:

$$F = \frac{\text{concentration of drug in the systemic circulation after oral administration}}{\text{concentration of drug in the systemic circulation after IV administration}}$$

    a. The **bioavailability** after oral administration depends on:
        (1) The **disintegration** of a tablet
        (2) The **dissolution** of the drug in the intestinal contents
        (3) Gastrointestinal and **first-pass metabolism**
    b. **Bioequivalence** occurs when drugs with equal F have the same drug concentration versus time relationship.

2. Apparent volume of distribution equation:

$$V_d = \frac{\text{amount of drug injected}}{\text{serum [drug]}}$$

    a. The V_d can be very large, even larger than the total body volume, if a drug is highly bound to tissues. This makes the serum drug concentration very low and the V_d very large.
    b. The V_d must be calculated at the time of injection.
    c. For the drugs illustrated in Figure 1–3, if the same amount of each was administered, the concentration of drug A at time 0 will be lower; thus, it will have the larger V_d.

3. The **loading dose** for a drug is based on the V_d.

$$\text{Oral loading dose} = \frac{V_d \times C}{F}$$

where C is the serum drug concentration.

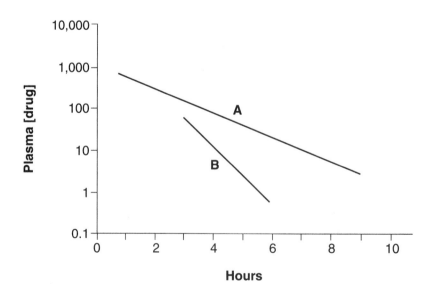

Figure 1-3. Relationship of plasma drug concentration versus time for two drugs. Drug A has the larger apparent volume of distribution.

4. **Clearance (Cl) equals $V_d \times K_e$**
  a. Clearance is measured as a volume per unit of time.
  b. The rate of drug elimination equals $Cl \times C_{ss}$, where C_{ss} is the drug concentration at steady state.
  c. The **oral maintenance dose** simply involves the replacement of the amount of drug that has been eliminated in the dosage interval (T)

$$\text{Oral maintenance dose} = \frac{Cl \times C_{ss} \times T}{F}$$

5. The **half-life** ($t_{1/2}$) of a drug is the time required for the serum drug concentration to be reduced by 50%.

  a. $t_{1/2} = \dfrac{0.69}{K_e}$

  b. If the $t_{1/2}$ of a drug is 5 hours, then the serum drug concentration will be reduced by 75% in 10 hours.
  c. During repeated administrations, it takes **4 to 5 half-lives to attain a steady state drug concentration.**
  d. When the dosage interval (T) is reduced with the same total amount of drug being administered, the $t_{1/2}$ is not changed.
    (1) The fluctuations of the drug concentration become smaller.
    (2) This is a useful approach when a drug has a very narrow therapeutic window between the effective drug concentration and the toxic drug concentration.

6. With **reduced kidney function,** the maintenance dose should be reduced if the drug is cleared from the body by the kidney.

  a. Oral maintenance dose $= \dfrac{(Cl_{hepatic} + Cl_{renal} + Cl_{others}) \times C_{ss} \times T}{F}$

  b. **Creatinine clearance** is a good quantitative **indicator of glomerular filtration rate.** Serum creatinine may also serve as a useful index of glomerular filtration rate.

7. With **reduced liver function,** there is **no good predictor** of the oral maintenance dose for drugs that are cleared by the liver.
  a. If the **extraction ratio** for a drug passing through the liver **approaches 1,** then Cl equals hepatic blood flow (BF).
    (1) **Reduced hepatic BF or reduced cardiac output (CO) will reduce the hepatic Cl of a drug with a high hepatic extraction ratio.**
    (2) An example is **lidocaine,** which has a lower $Cl_{hepatic}$ in patients with congestive heart failure. As a result, the maintenance dose of lidocaine should be reduced in these patients.
  b. If the hepatic extraction ratio is near 0, hepatic BF is unimportant. Intrinsic metabolic rate and the amount of plasma protein binding become important factors.

8. If a drug follows first-order elimination kinetics, **doubling the dose will double the C_{ss}.**

E. The above equations **do not apply** to drugs that have **zero-order** elimination kinetics (i.e., those for which a constant amount of drug is eliminated per unit of time).

1. It is very difficult to predict and control the C_{ss} for these drugs.

2. Drugs which follow zero-order kinetics include:
   a. Ethanol
   b. Heparin
   c. Phenytoin
   d. Aspirin at high concentrations

V. PEDIATRIC PHARMACOLOGY

A. Newborns have **more body water and less body fat** than adults.

   1. A **water-soluble drug will have a higher** V_d (relative to body size) in children than in adults.

   2. A **lipid-soluble drug will have a lower** V_d (relative to body size) in children than in adults.

B. **Plasma protein binding is reduced** for approximately the first year.

C. **Metabolism,** especially oxidation and glucuronidation, is also **reduced** in the newborn.

D. **Glomerular filtration rate (GFR) and renal tubular function** are **reduced** in newborns.

VI. GERIATRIC PHARMACOLOGY

A. The **elderly** generally have:

   1. A **smaller** body mass

   2. **More body fat** and less body water
      a. A water soluble drug will have a lower V_d than in a person of average age.
      b. A lipid soluble drug will have a higher V_d.

   3. **Reduced plasma albumin,** which will reduce the amount of bound drug in the plasma

   4. **Reduced renal excretion**

   5. **Reduced hepatic metabolism** of some drugs

   6. Other non-pharmacokinetic changes
      a. Central nervous system (CNS) drugs often produce confusion.
      b. Cardiovascular drugs often have greater effects in the elderly patient because the homeostatic mechanisms (e.g., baroreceptor reflexes) are sluggish.

B. Overall, elderly patients require smaller dosages of most drugs than young adults.

VII. PHARMACODYNAMICS

A. **Pharmacodynamics** is a description of the properties of **drug-receptor interactions.**

B. **Drugs bind** to specific receptors with:

   1. Ionic bonds

   2. Hydrogen bonds

   3. Van der Waals forces, which are weak but necessary for a good fit

   4. Covalent bonds, which are uncommon and are usually irreversible

C. **Agonists** change the effector site and **lead to drug effects.**

    1. The drug-receptor interaction follows the **laws of mass action.**

        a. Drug molecules bind to receptors at a rate that is dependent on the drug concentration.

        b. The number of drug-receptor interactions determines the magnitude of the drug effect.

    2. This leads to **dose–response** curves, which can be:

        a. **Quantal** (all or none) [e.g., death]

        b. **Graded** (e.g., blood pressure)

D. The **therapeutic index** (TI) is a measure of the **safety** of a drug. (Figure 1–4)

$$TI = \frac{LD_{50}}{ED_{50}}$$

    1. LD_{50} is the dose that kills 50% of the subjects.

    2. ED_{50} is the dose that produces the desired effect in 50% of the subjects.

E. Other indexes can be used, including:

    1. $\dfrac{LD_1}{ED_{99}}$

    2. $\dfrac{TD_{50}}{ED_{50}}$, where TD_{50} is the dose that induces a toxic effect in 50% of the subjects.

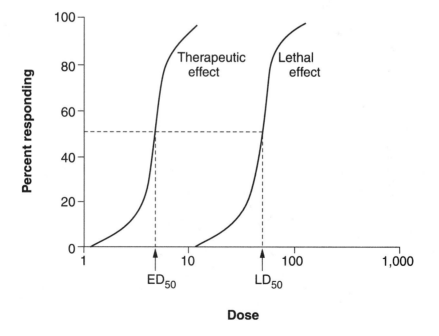

Figure 1-4. Dose-response relationships for a therapeutic effect and the lethal effect of a drug. The distance between these curves is indicative of the safety of the drug and the TI is approximately 10. ED_{50} = effective dose in 50% of patients; LD_{50} = lethal dose in 50% of patients

F. The **potency** (affinity) of a drug is inversely related to the ED_{50}.

G. The **intrinsic activity** (efficacy) is equivalent to the **maximal effect.**

    1. In Figure 1–5, drug B has the higher intrinsic activity.

    2. Drug A (See Figure 1–5) is approximately 10 times more potent than drug B, because the ED_{50} of drug A is 10% the ED_{50} of drug B.

    3. Drug A is a partial agonist (or a partial antagonist), because the maximal response is smaller.

H. **Antagonists** are drugs with a high affinity for a receptor and **no intrinsic activity.** They alter the dose-response curves for the agonists.

    1. **Competitive surmountable** (reversible) antagonists induce a **parallel shift** of the agonist dose-response curve to the right with no change in intrinsic activity (Figure 1–6A). In other words, the effect of the antagonist can be surmounted by increasing the concentration of the agonist.

    2. The **maximal effect** of a specific agonist **is reduced** (increasing the concentration of the agonist will not surmount the effect of the antagonist) with little or no change in the ED_{50} of the agonist (Figure 1–6B) by:

        a. **Competitive insurmountable (irreversible) antagonists,** which often bind covalently to a receptor

        b. **Non-competitive antagonists,** which often act at a site other than the receptor for the agonist

I. **Other types of antagonism** can occur.

    1. **Functional** (physiological) antagonism involves the opposing actions of **2 agonists** at different receptors [e.g., acetylcholine (ACh) and norepinephrine (NE) on heart rate].

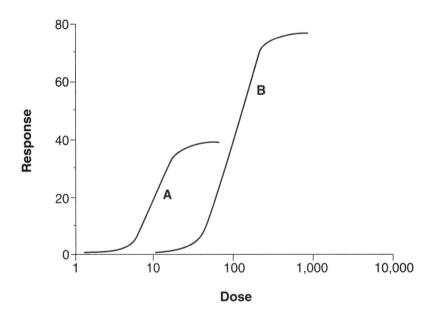

Figure 1-5. Dose-response relationships for two drugs. Drug B has the higher intrinsic activity. Drug A is approximately 10 times more potent than Drug B.

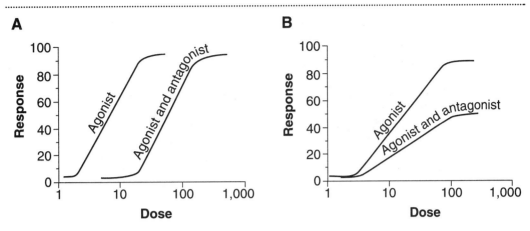

Figure 1-6. Dose-response relationships for an agonist alone and for an agonist in the presence of (A) a competitive surmountable antagonist and (B) a competitive insurmountable or non-competitive antagonist.

Table 1-1
Procedures for Development of New Drugs (established by Kefauver-Harris Amendment, 1962)

1. **Animal studies** are initially performed to determine the activity and toxicity in more than one species.
2. An **IND application** is submitted to the FDA.
3. The **clinical phases** are begun.
   - **Phase 1** involves studies of kinetics in approximately 10 healthy volunteers.
   - **Phase 2** involves studies of the dosage range, effectiveness and toxicity in approximately 100 patients, utilizing single or double-blind methods.
   - **Phase 3** involves studies of the same parameters in approximately 1000 patients. Special attention is paid to toxicities with low frequencies.
   - The **NDA** must be approved by the FDA.
   - **Phase 4** (NDA Phase) is a monitored release of the new drug to many physicians to detect rare toxicities.

FDA=Food and Drug Administration; IND=Investigational New Drug; NDA=New Drug Application

    2. **Chemical antagonism** involves the **direct binding** of a drug by another drug without the involvement of a receptor (e.g., heavy metal chelators).

VIII. REGULATIONS GOVERNING THE DEVELOPMENT OF NEW DRUGS

A. In 1962, the **Kefauver-Harris Amendment to the Food, Drug and Cosmetic Act of 1938** was passed, as a result of thalidomide toxicity that occurred in Europe.

    1. The **Food and Drug Administration (FDA)** was charged with regulating drugs.

    2. **Procedures** were developed **for testing** new drugs. The procedures include animal studies, an Investigational New Drug (IND) application, human studies, and a New Drug Application (NDA) (Table 1–1).

B. The **ANDA** (Abbreviated NDA) was established so that it is only necessary to demonstrate bioequivalence for a generic form of an approved drug.

C. **Prescriptions** are required to dispense drugs that are:

1. **In the NDA Phase** of development

2. **Toxic**

3. **Habit-forming.** These drugs are divided into schedules based on their **potential for abuse.**
   a. **Schedule C-I drugs** are abused drugs with **no clinical use.**
   b. The others are **clinically useful.**
      (1) **Schedule C-II** drugs are highly abused.
      (2) **Schedule C-III** drugs are less commonly abused.
      (3) **Schedule C-IV** drugs are even less commonly abused.
      (4) **Schedule C-V** drugs have minor potential for abuse and may even be available over-the-counter.

2

Peripheral Neuropharmacology

I. OVERVIEW OF THE AUTONOMIC NERVOUS SYSTEM

A. This part of the peripheral nervous system **regulates the activity of cardiac muscle, smooth muscle,** and **exocrine glands.** It has two major divisions.

1. The **parasympathetic nervous system** refers to the division of the autonomic nervous system arising from the **brainstem** and the **sacral region** of the spinal cord.

a. **Acetylcholine (ACh)** is the neurotransmitter at **both the ganglionic and neuroeffector synapses** (Figure 2–1).

b. The **receptors** activated by ACh in the ganglion are **nicotinic (N) cholinoceptors,** and those in the neuroeffector junction are **muscarinic (M) cholinoceptors.**

2. The **sympathetic nervous system** refers to the division of the autonomic nervous system arising from the **thoracic and lumbar** regions of the spinal cord.

a. **ACh** is the neurotransmitter in the **ganglionic synapse;** and **norepinephrine (NE)** is the neurotransmitter at the **neuroeffector synapse. Exceptions** include:

(1) N-cholinergic innervation of the **adrenal medulla**

(2) Sympathetic M-cholinergic innervation of some **sweat glands**

(3) Sympathetic M-cholinergic innervation of some **muscle blood vessels**

(4) Sympathetic dopaminergic innervation of **renal blood vessels**

b. The **receptors** in the ganglion are **N-cholinoceptors** and those at the neuroeffector junction are **α- and β-adrenoceptors.**

B. The **synthesis and breakdown** of the **neurotransmitters** in the autonomic nervous system have been determined.

1. ACh is synthesized in the nerve terminal from **choline and acetyl coenzyme A in the presence of choline acetyltransferase.** After it is released, the ACh is broken down to choline and acetate by cholinesterases.

2. NE synthesis involves many steps (Figure 2–2).

a. **Tyrosine hydroxylase** is the **rate-limiting step** in the synthesis and is also the **site for negative feedback inhibition** by NE.

b. **Dopamine (DA)** is taken up into the granule and **metabolized by the granular enzyme, DA β-hydroxylase.**

c. NE is complexed to adenosine triphosphate (ATP) and chromogranin in the granule.

d. **Sites where epinephrine (EPI) is a neurotransmitter** have a **methyltransferase** that **converts NE to EPI.**

Parasympathetic transmitters (cranial and sacral)

Sympathetic transmitters (thoracic and lumbar)

Figure 2-1. Neurotransmitters in the parasympathetic and sympathetic nervous systems. N = nicotinic cholinoceptors, M = muscarinic cholinoceptors, α = α-adrenoceptors, β = β-adrenoceptors. *ACh*=acetylcholine; *NE*=norepinephrine

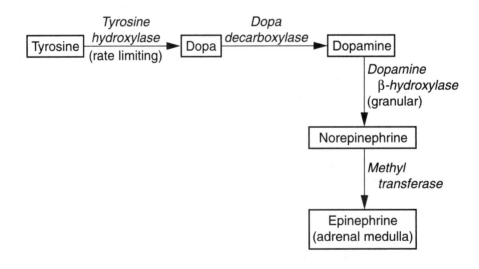

Figure 2-2. Synthesis of norepinephrine.

    e. The NE that is released **can be taken back up into the nerve ending (reuptake),** it can be **metabolized,** or it can **diffuse away from the synapse.**

      (1) **Reuptake** is the most important mechanism for the termination of NE action.

      (2) **Cocaine** or **tricyclic antidepressants block the reuptake** of NE, thereby enhancing the neurotransmitter effects.

    f. **Catechol-O-methyltransferase (COMT)** and **monoamine oxidase (MAO)** convert NE to a final product, **methoxyhydroxymandelic acid (vanillylmandelic acid)** that **accounts for 90% of the NE and NE metabolites found in the urine** (Figure 2–3).

C. The **effects of sympathetic and parasympathetic nerve stimulation** are listed in Table 2–1. Many of the effects of the autonomic drugs can be predicted from a thorough understanding of this table.

II. PARASYMPATHOMIMETICS

A. Drugs in this class produce effects similar to activation of the parasympathetic nervous system.

B. Specific drugs

    1. **ACh** acts at **N-cholinoceptors** and **M-cholinoceptors.**

      a. There are **2 binding sites** for ACh on the ACh receptors. One binds the **quaternary nitrogen** and the second binds the **carbonyl oxygen** (Figure 2–4).

      b. ACh has some major **disadvantages.**

        (1) It **activates all cholinoceptors, which are present in most internal organs,** leading to **many side effects** from administration.

        (2) It has a **short duration of action** due to rapid metabolism by cholinesterases.

    2. **Analogues of ACh** are available that have slightly different properties than ACh (Table 2–2)

      a. All of these are **quaternary ammonium** compounds.

      b. **Carbachol** and **bethanechol** have **greater effects on the gastrointestinal** and **urinary tracts** and **longer durations of action** than ACh and methacholine.

    3. **Two alkaloids** have parasympathomimetic activity.

      a. **Muscarine** is a **quaternary amine** that acts only on muscarinic receptors.

      b. **Pilocarpine** is a **tertiary amine** that acts only on muscarinic receptors.

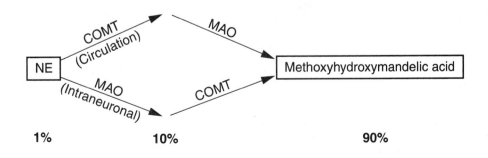

Figure 2-3. Metabolism of norepinephrine by catechol-O-methyl transferase (COMT) and monoamine oxidase (MAO). The percentages represent the proportions of each form found in the urine. *NE*=norepinephrine

(1) As a tertiary amine, it is **more readily absorbed.**

(2) It **penetrates the blood-brain barrier** to reach the CNS.

C. The effects of all the parasympathomimetics are **similar to the effects of parasympathetic nerve stimulation** (see Table 2–1).

    1. The parasympathomimetics also **activate uninnervated cholinoceptors** (e.g., M-cholinoceptors in blood vessels) and M-cholinoceptors at sympathetic cholinergic synapses.

    2. The effects of parasympathomimetics **on blood vessels are mediated by the release of endothelium-derived relaxing factor (EDRF),** which is probably nitric

Table 2-1
Effects of Autonomic Nerve Activity on Organ Function

Organ	Sympathetic Nerve Activity	Parasympathetic Nerve Activity
Eye	α-contracts radial muscle (mydriasis)	M-contracts circular muscle (miosis)
	—	M-contracts ciliary muscle
Heart	β_1-accelerates SA node	M-decelerates SA node
	β_1-accelerates conduction	M-decelerates conduction
	β_1-increases contractility	—
Vascular smooth muscle	α-constricts skin and splanchnic vessels	—M(+)
	β_2-dilates skeletal muscle vessels	
	M-dilates skeletal muscle vessels (minor)	
	DA-dilates renal and mesenteric vessels	
Bronchiolar smooth muscle	β_2-dilates bronchioles	M-constricts bronchioles
Gastrointestinal tract	β_2-reduces gut contractility	M-increases gut contractility
	α-contracts sphincters	M-relaxes sphincters
	—	M-increases secretions
Genitourinary tract	β_2-reduces bladder motility	M-increases bladder motility
	α-contracts sphincters	M-relaxes sphincters
	β_2-relaxes the pregnant uterus	—
	α-contracts the uterus	—
	α-ejaculation	M-penile erection
Skin	α-contracts pilomotor smooth muscle	—
	M-induces sweating	—
Metabolic functions	α, β_2-increases hepatic gluconeogenesis	—
	α, β_2-increases hepatic glycogenolysis	—
	β_1-increases lipolysis	—
Glands	α_1-thick salivary secretions	M-thin salivary secretions
	—	M-lacrimal and respiratory secretions
Adrenal gland	N-secretes EPI and NE	—
	β_1-increases renin release	—

+ Most blood vessels have uninnervated muscarinic cholinoceptors. Relaxation involves release of endothelium-derived relaxing factor (EDRF) from the endothelium.

α=α-adrenoceptors; β=β-adrenocepters; DA=dopamine; EPI=epinephrine; M=muscarinic cholinoceptors; N=nicotinic cholinoceptors; NE=nonepinephrine; SA=sinoatrial; — = no effect

Figure 2-4. Binding of acetylcholine to the cholinoceptor. The two bars represent the binding sites on the receptor.

Table 2-2
Properties of ACh and ACh analogues

	Metabolized by cholinesterases	Nicotinic activity	GI activity	CV activity
ACh	+++	+	++	+++
Methacholine	+	⊖	+	⟨+++⟩
Carbachol	⊖	+	⟨+++⟩	+
Bethanechol (*Urecholine*)	⊖	⊖	⟨+++⟩	+

Note: unique features are circled
ACh=acetylcholine; *CV*=cardiovascular; *GI*=gastrointestinal

oxide, from the endothelium. An intact endothelium is required for these effects to occur.

3. An **overdose** of a parasympathomimetic leads to:
   a. **A marked fall in blood pressure**
   b. **An increase in heart rate,** mediated via **reflexes** induced by the fall in blood pressure. The fall in blood pressure reduces the baroreceptor activity which leads to an increase in efferent sympathetic tone to the heart.
   c. Activation of M-cholinoceptors at many sites which induces a **DUMBELS syndrome,** composed of
   (1) Defecation
   (2) Urination
   (3) Miosis
   (4) Bronchoconstriction
   (5) Emesis
   (6) Lacrimation
   (7) Salivation

D. The **clinical uses** of the parasympathomimetics are **limited.**
   1. **Gastrointestinal (GI) atony and bladder atony** can be treated with bethanechol.
   2. **Glaucoma** can be treated with pilocarpine.
   3. A **pupillary constriction** can be induced with pilocarpine.
   4. A **diagnosis of atropine poisoning or asthma** can utilize methacholine.

III. CHOLINESTERASE INHIBITORS

A. These drugs bind to and **inhibit acetylcholinesterases,** thereby **increasing the ACh concentration** in the cholinergic synapses.

1. Cholinesterase inhibitors are **indirect parasympathomimetics** because they **do not bind to ACh receptors.**

2. Butyrylcholinesterases (pseudocholinesterases) are also inhibited by the cholinesterase inhibitors, but the function of these cholinesterases is unknown.

3. The **characteristics of the important cholinesterase inhibitors** are summarized in Table 2–3 .

4. The mechanism of binding to cholinesterase varies, as **some bind both the esteratic (E) and anionic (A) sites,** and **some bind only one site** (See Table 2–3).

B. The **carbamates** and **edrophonium** are **reversible inhibitors** of cholinesterases.

C. The quaternary amines will not induce CNS effects because the quaternary structure precludes passage across the blood-brain barrier.

D. The **organophosphates** are **very lipid soluble** and are **irreversible inhibitors of cholinesterases.** This group includes

1. Diisopropyl phosphorofluoridate (DFP)

2. Echothiophate (*Phospholine*)

3. **Malathion** and **parathion**
a. They must be metabolized to their active forms, **malaoxan** and **paraoxan.**
b. They are more toxic to insects than to humans, because humans detoxify them more rapidly.

E. Effects

1. The effects of the cholinesterase inhibitors are primarily **muscarinic** in nature.
a. A **DUMBELS** syndrome is induced.
b. **Nicotinic effects** occur **only at high doses.**

2. An **overdose of cholinesterase inhibitors** causes **death** from **respiratory insufficiency.**
a. The reduced respiratory function is due to
(1) Increased bronchial secretions
(2) Bronchoconstriction
(3) Central respiratory depression
(4) Depolarizing neuromuscular blockade
b. The **specific antidotes** used for poisoning by the cholinesterase inhibitors are:
(1) **Atropine at high dosages,** which blocks the muscarinic effects of the accumulated ACh.
(2) **Pralidoxime (2-PAM)** (*Protopam*) which can **reactivate the cholinesterases** that have been inhibited by an organophosphate.

Table 2-3
Properties of Various Cholinesterase Inhibitors

Inhibitor	Binding sites	Chemical properties
Physostigmine (*Antilirium*)	E & A	Tertiary carbamate
Neostigmine (*Prostigmin*)	E & A	Quaternary carbamate
Pyridostigmine (*Mestinon*)	E & A	Quaternary carbamate
Edrophonium (*Tensilon*)	A	Quaternary (non-carbamate), short duration
Organophospates	E	Irreversible

A=anionic; *E*=esteratic

(a) It **must be administered within a few hours after the exposure,** because an "aging" process occurs, and the organophosphate-cholinesterase complex becomes insensitive to 2-PAM.

(b) Pralidoxime will have **no effect on poisoning from the carbamates.**

3. Chronic exposure to the organophosphates leads to a **delayed neurotoxicity** due to **demyelinization of motor neurons.**

F. These drugs have many **clinical uses.**

1. Paroxysmal supraventricular tachycardia (PSVT) can be terminated with edrophonium.

2. Glaucoma can be reduced with echothiophate.

3. Competitive neuromuscular blockade can be reversed with neostigmine.
  a. To **reduce the parasympathetic side effects of the cholinesterase inhibitors, atropine** should also be administered.
  b. Atropine has no effect on the skeletal neuromuscular junction, because there are no M-cholinoceptors at this site.

4. Myasthenia gravis is treated with pyridostigmine.

5. Myasthenia gravis can be diagnosed, and a **myasthenic crisis** can be differentiated from a **cholinergic crisis** with edrophonium.

6. Alzheimer's disease can be somewhat reduced with tacrine (*Cognex*).

7. Anticholinergic poisoning can be treated with cholinesterase inhibitors.

G. Contraindications for the use of cholinesterase inhibitors include:

1. Asthma

2. Peptic ulcers

IV. PARASYMPATHETIC BLOCKING DRUGS

A. Drugs in this class **block the effects of the parasympathetic nervous system.**

1. Atropine is a **competitive, surmountable antagonist.**
  a. It blocks M_1, M_2, and M_3 cholinoreceptors.
  b. The **effects of ACh are reversed** (ACh reversal) by muscarinic antagonists.
    (1) The **muscarinic vasodilating actions** of ACh are **blocked.**
    (2) The **nicotinic (ganglion) vasoconstricting actions** from high doses of ACh are **unmasked.**
  c. At very high concentrations (1000 times), atropine has local anesthetic activity.

2. Scopolamine is similar to atropine, except there are more CNS effects, which may occur even at therapeutic doses.

3. Both are **tertiary amines,** so they will penetrate into the CNS.

B. The **effects, uses,** and **side effects** are summarized in Table 2–4. Note that atropine will not increase blood pressure because there is no parasympathetic tone to the blood vessels.

C. Both anticholinergics and phenylephrine, an α_1-adrenoceptor agonist, induce mydriasis, but **phenylephrine will not induce cycloplegia** (loss of accommodation).

D. These drugs have a **large therapeutic index.**

1. Hallucinations can be induced.

Table 2-4

Effects, Uses, and Side Effects of the Parasympathetic Blocking Drugs

Effects	Uses	Side effects
Increase heart rate (may be an initial decrease due to vagal nuclei activity)	Bradycardia with hypotension (e.g., digoxin therapy)	Tachycardia
Pupillary dilation and cycloplegia	Eye exam [tropicamide (*Mydriacyl*)]	Blurred vision Photophobia Angle closure glaucoma
Bronchodilation	Asthma [quarternary: ipratropium (*Atrovent*)]	
Decrease gut motility	Antispasmodic [propantheline (*Pro-Banthine*)]	Constipation
Decrease bladder contractions		Urinary retention
Decrease secretions	Preanesthetic medication	Dry mouth
Sedative	Preanesthetic medication	Drowsiness (scopolamine)
	Reduce motion sickness (scopolamine)	
	Parkinson's disease [trihexyphenidyl (*Artane*)]	
	Antagonize poisoning from cholinesterase inhibitors and muscarine	

   2. High doses produce **life-threatening toxicity only in children,** who seem to be more sensitive to the drugs.

   a. The side effects in Table 2–4 will be accentuated.

   b. Hot skin and fever occur, due to a direct vasodilation.

   3. Adult anticholinergic poisoning is more common with H_1 antihistamines, tricyclic antidepressants, and phenothiazines.

   4. The antidote for anticholinergic poisoning is a **cholinesterase inhibitor** (e.g., physostigmine).

V. GANGLIONIC BLOCKING DRUGS

   A. Drugs in this class **competitively inhibit nicotinic cholinoceptors in the ganglion,** which leads to ganglionic blockade. These drugs have no effect on the neuromuscular nicotinic cholinoceptors.

   1. Hexamethonium and **trimethaphan** (*Arfonad*) are **polar amines.**

   2. Trimethaphan has a very short duration of action and is thus useful to treat hypertensive crises.

   B. The **major limitation** of the ganglionic blocking drugs is that they **inhibit both sympathetic and parasympathetic ganglia.**

   1. This results in **many autonomic side effects.**

   2. More selective drugs are available for the treatment of **essential hypertension.**

   C. When both sympathetic and parasympathetic ganglia are blocked by hexamethonium, the net effect will be equivalent to blockade of the dominant autonomic system for each tissue.

    D. Nicotine activates nicotinic receptors at:

        1. Sensory nerve endings

        2. Ganglia

        3. Adrenal medulla

        4. **Neuromuscular junction,** leading to depolarization block

VI. SYMPATHOMIMETICS

    A. Drugs in this class **mimic the effects of the sympathetic nervous system** by activating adrenoceptors or inducing the release of endogenous NE.

    B. There are 2 groups of sympathomimetics.

        1. **Catecholamines** have a **catechol** (3,4 dihydroxybenzine) in the structure (Figure 2–5).

            a. The *l*-form is active.

            b. **Administration by parenteral injection or inhalation** is used because of metabolism in the gut and first-pass metabolism.

            c. Important **catecholamines** are:

                (1) NE, an α and β_1 agonist

                (2) EPI, an α, β_1 and β_2 agonist

                (3) Isoproterenol (Iso), a β_1 and β_2 agonist

                (4) DA, which:

                    (a) Is an agonist at **DA receptors (vasodilates renal and mesenteric blood vessels)** at low doses

                    (b) Is an **indirect agonist** and a β_1 agonist at intermediate doses

                    (c) Is an α agonist at high doses

        2. **Phenylethylamines** do not have the catechol structure and thus are **less readily metabolized** and **more effective when given orally.**

            a. **Phenylephrine** (*Neo-Synephrine*) and methoxamine (*Vasoxyl*) are α_1 agonists.

            b. **Clonidine** (*Catapres*) is an α_2 agonist.

            c. **Dobutamine** (*Dobutrex*) is a β_1 agonist.

            d. **Terbutaline** (*Bricanyl, Brethine*) and **albuterol** (*Proventil, Ventolin*) are β_2 agonists.

            e. **Tyramine** and the **amphetamines** are **indirect** sympathomimetics.

                (1) This means that they induce the release of endogeneous NE and it is the NE that activates the α- and β-adrenoceptors.

                (2) **Effects** of the indirect sympathomimetics will be **reduced by the following procedures.** The same procedures will not affect or will increase the effects of the direct sympathomimetics.

                3,4 Dihydroxybenzine   **Ethylamine**
                      (catechol)

Figure 2-5. General structure of catecholamines, as illustrated with NE.

(a) **Cocaine and tricyclic antidepressants** block the uptake of tyramine and NE into the adrenergic nerve ending, an action that reduces the effect of tyramine and augments the effects of exogenously administered NE.

(b) **Denervation, reserpine and guanethidine** deplete the endogenous catecholamines, thus the indirect agonists become ineffective and the effects of exogenous NE will be unchanged or enhanced.

C. The **cardiovascular effects** of each agonist will depend on the types of receptors that are activated.

1. α_1-**Agonists** will induce (Figure 2–6):

   a. An **increase in blood pressure**

   b. A **reflex reduction in heart rate.** This also occurs with NE, indicating that the reflex effects are more important than the direct effects on the heart.

2. β-**Agonists** will induce (Figure 2–7):

   a. A **decrease in blood pressure (β_2)**

   b. **Large increases in heart rate and contractility,** due to both direct (β_1) and reflex effects.

Figure 2-6. Effects of α-adrenoceptor activation on blood pressure and heart rate. The reflex effects on the heart (blocked by atropine) will predominate over the direct beta effects, if norepinephrine is the agonist.

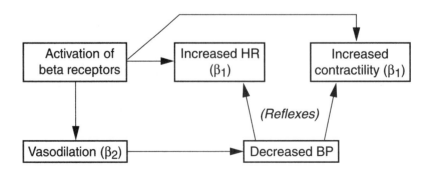

Figure 2-7. Effects of β-adrenoceptor activation on blood pressure and heart rate. Both the reflex and direct effects result in an increase in heart rate and contractility. *BP*=blood pressure; *HR*=heart rate

D. Many of the effects of the catecholamines, especially the β-effects, are mediated by the second messenger, **cyclic adenosine monophosphate (cAMP).**

E. The **effects, uses,** and **side effects** for the various sympathomimetics are summarized in Table 2–5.

VII. α-ADRENOCEPTOR ANTAGONISTS

A. Drugs in this class **inhibit α-adrenoceptors,** thereby **reducing the α-effects of endogenously released NE.**

B. **Non-selective** antagonists block both α_1- and α_2-adrenoceptors.

    1. The properties of the various α-antagonists are quite different.

        a. **Phenoxybenzamine** (*Dibenzyline*) is an **alkylating agent** due to the formation of a reactive intermediate.

            (1) A **covalent** (irreversible) interaction with α-receptors results in a **competitive, insurmountable antagonism.**

            (2) Phenoxybenzamine is very irritating when given subcutaneously or intramuscularly and therefore **can only be given orally** or **intravenously.**

        b. **Phentolamine** (*Regitine*) is a **competitive, surmountable antagonist.**

            (1) The **duration of action is short.**

            (2) It is effective after oral or parenteral administration.

        c. **Ergot alkaloids** are α-antagonists, vasoconstrictors, and oxytocics.

            (1) **Ergotoxine** is the most potent **α-antagonist.**

            (2) **Ergotamine** is the most potent **vasoconstrictor.** The vasoconstriction is unrelated to autonomic receptor actions.

Table 2-5
Effects, Uses, and Side Effects from Activation of Adrenergic Receptors

Receptors	Effects	Uses	Side effects
α	Vasoconstriction	Hypotension Nasal congestion Reduce bleeding PSVT (phenylephrine) Prolong local anesthesia (EPI)	Hypertension Ischemia Bradycardia
β_1	Increased myocardial contractility	Cardiac arrest (Iso and dobutamine)	Coronary insufficiency Palpitations
β_1	Increased myocardial conduction	Heart block	Tachycardia Arrhythmias
β_2	Bronchodilation	Anaphylactic shock (EPI) Asthma (Iso, terbutaline and albuterol)	Muscle tremor
β_1	Increased cardiac output	Cardiogenic shock (DA)	
DA	Dilated renal and mesenteric vessels		
β_2	Uterine relaxation	Premature labor (ritodrine)	
α	Mydriasis without cycloplegia	Eye exam (phenylephrine)	
	Reduced intraocular pressure	Glaucoma (EPI)	

DA=dopamine; *EPI*=epinephrine; *Iso*=isoproterenol; *PVST*=paroxysmal supraventricular tachycardia

(3) Ergonovine is the most potent **oxytocic.**

2. When EPI is administered IV in the presence of an α-antagonist, the **normal pressor effect of EPI is reversed to a depressor effect.**

    a. α-Receptor activation by EPI, which normally increases blood pressure, is blocked.

    b. β_2-Receptor activation by EPI leads to a drop of blood pressure.

3. The effect of NE on blood pressure is inhibited, but not reversed, by the α-antagonists, because NE has much weaker β-agonistic effects than EPI.

4. The clinical **uses** of phenoxybenzamine and phentolamine are limited.

    a. **Pheochromocytoma** can be diagnosed and treated.

    b. **Peripheral vascular disease** can be treated.

    c. Blood pressure is reduced, but not by very much; thus they are **not used to treat essential hypertension.** Also, **side effects** are more common than with other anti-hypertensive drugs.

        (1) **Postural hypotension** results from:

            (a) **Venule dilation**

            (b) **Impaired sympathetic reflexes** to the blood vessels

        (2) **Tachycardia** results from increased sympathetic reflexes to the heart. This effect is enhanced by the α_2-blockade (blockade of presynaptic inhibitory sites), which leads to increased NE release and increased NE effects at sites where β-receptors predominate (e.g., myocardium).

        (3) **Renin release is increased.**

C. The newer drugs are **selective α-antagonists.**

    1. **Prazosin** (*Minipress*), **doxazosin** (*Cardura*) and **terazosin** (*Hytrin*) are selective α_1-antagonists.

        a. Blood pressure is reduced with less tachycardia and less renin release than with the non-selective antagonists.

        b. **Clinical indications** include:

            (1) **Essential hypertension**

            (2) **Prostatic hypertrophy**

        c. An important **side effect** is **first-dose syncope.**

    2. **Yohimbine** is a selective α_2-**antagonist** with no demonstrated clinical usefulness.

VIII. β-ADRENOCEPTOR ANTAGONISTS

A. Drugs in this class **inhibit β-adrenoceptors,** thereby **reducing the β-effects of endogenously released NE.**

B. β-Blockers are **structurally similar to the catecholamines.**

    1. They have **bulky alkyl** substitutions on the nitrogen and an **oxymethylene bridge** near the aromatic ring.

    2. The *l*-isomers are the active forms.

C. The non-selective β-blockers inhibit both β_1- and β_2-adrenoceptors.

    1. **Propranolol** (*Inderal*) is 90% bound to plasma proteins and is **rapidly metabolized** by the liver.

        a. The bioavailability is low (F = 0.3) due to first pass metabolism.

        b. The IV dose is one third of the oral dose.

        c. The half-life is short, approximately 3 hours.

        d. An active metabolite, hydroxypropranolol, is formed.

2. The **effects, uses, side effects,** and **contraindications** of the β-blockers (e.g., propranolol) are listed in Table 2–6.

3. Other **non-selective β-blockers** have important differences from propranolol.
  a. **Nadolol** (*Corgard*) is non-selective, water soluble and not metabolized, so the **half-life is long** (15 hours).
  b. **Pindolol** (*Visken*) is non-selective with **intrinsic sympathomimetic activity (ISA).**
    (1) It is a partial antagonist with β-agonistic activity.
    (2) Drugs with ISA induce less bradycardia.
  c. **Labetalol** (*Normodyne, Trandate*) is non-selective with **α-blocking activity.** It decreases blood pressure with less change of heart rate and contractility than other β-blockers.

D. **Selective β$_1$-blockers (cardioselective)** have weaker actions on the bronchi, making them more useful in patients with **asthma.** The β$_1$-selectivity is relative, however, so these drugs can still be dangerous when administered to asthmatics.

  1. **Metoprolol** (*Lopressor*) is β$_1$-selective.

  2. **Atenolol** (*Tenormin*) is β$_1$-selective and **water soluble,** which results in **fewer CNS effects.**

  3. **Acebutolol** (*Sectral*) is β$_1$-selective with **ISA.**

  4. **Esmolol** (*Brevibloc*) is β$_1$-selective and is rapidly metabolized by esterases (**t$_{1/2}$ = 9 minutes),** making it useful for emergency therapy.

Table 2-6
Effects, Uses, Side Effects, and Contraindications of Beta-Blockers

Effects	Uses	Side effects	Contraindications
Decreased heart rate	Tachycardia Angina Hyperthyroid crisis	Bradycardia	
Prolonged AV conduction time	Arrhythmias (e.g. PSVT)	Slow AV conduction	Heart block
Decreased myocardial contractility	Angina	Congestive heart failure	Congestive heart failure
Bronchoconstriction		Bronchospasm	Asthma
Decreased glycogenolysis		Hypoglycemia	Diabetes
Peripheral vasoconstriction		Vasoconstriction	Peripheral vascular disease Angina at rest
Decreased blood pressure	Hypertension		
	Glaucoma Migraine		
		CNS depression Insomnia Nightmares Sudden withdrawal can increase BP and induce arrhythmias	

AV=atrioventricular; *BP*=blood pressure; *CNS*=central nervous system; *PSVT*=paroxysmal supraventricular tachycardia

IX. ADRENERGIC NEURON BLOCKING DRUGS

A. These drugs have **no adrenoceptor blocking effects.** Instead, they **reduce the release of NE from the postganglionic adrenergic neuron.**

B. **Reserpine** (*Serpasil*) **depletes monoamines** [NE, DA and serotonin (5-HT)] and the depletion of NE results in a lowering of blood pressure.

   1. It acts by blocking the **granular catecholamine uptake.** Neuronal catecholamine uptake is unaffected.

   2. The **side effects** are very marked, including:

      a. **Profound psychological depression and sedation.** It must be used with caution when treating patients with a history of depression.

      b. **Extrapyramidal symptoms** from DA depletion

C. **Guanethidine** (*Ismelin*) is transported to the site of action in the nerve terminal via the neuronal catecholamine transport mechanism. The effects are **blocked by uptake inhibitors** (e.g., cocaine and tricyclic antidepressants).

   1. There is an **initial release of NE.**

   2. The **release is subsequently reduced** and depletion also occurs.

   3. The drug is very effective; but has **prominent side effects,** including:

      a. Symptoms of severe sympathetic block

      b. Severe postural hypotension

      c. Marked impotence

      d. Severe diarrhea

D. Several drugs **act on the CNS** to reduce the efferent sympathetic tone to the cardiovascular system.

   1. **Methyldopa** (*Aldomet*) is metabolized in CNS adrenergic neurons to **α-methyldopamine and α-methylnorepinephrine (α-methylNE).**

      a. α-MethylNE acts on α_2-adrenoceptors and decreases the sympathetic outflow from the medulla.

      b. The site of action appears to be the **nucleus tractus solitarius.**

   2. **Clonidine** (*Catapres*) and **guanabenz** (*Wytensin*) are α_2-**adrenoceptor agonists** that act like α-methylNE in the medulla.

   3. Side effects from the CNS active sympathetic blockers include:

      a. Drowsiness

      b. Fluid retention

      c. Positive Coombs' test (increased risk for hemolytic anemia) with **methyldopa**

      d. Acute withdrawal hypertension with clonidine

E. **Bretylium** (*Bretylol*) decreases NE release and is used for cardiac arrhythmias.

F. α-**Methyltyrosine** competitively **inhibits tyrosine hydroxylase,** which depletes the NE. It is used to treat **pheochromocytoma,** if surgery is not possible.

X. DRUGS FOR GLAUCOMA

A. **Open angle glaucoma** is the most common type. It is treated with:

   1. **Pilocarpine** to **increase outflow** of intraocular fluid

   2. **Timolol** (*Timoptic*), a β-blocker, to **reduce the production** of intraocular fluid

   3. **EPI** to both increase outflow and reduce production of intraocular fluid

B. **Angle closure glaucoma** is induced when the iris dilates and obstructs the drainage of intraocular fluid. **Antimuscarinics,** which are pupillary dilators, can induce this type of glaucoma.

1. Pilocarpine will **constrict the pupil** and lower the intraocular pressure.

2. **Osmotic agents** will draw fluid from the eye.

3. **Surgery** can correct the defect.

XI. NEUROMUSCULAR BLOCKING DRUGS

A. Drugs in this class **block skeletal neuromuscular transmission, thereby inducing a paralysis.**

B. **Competitive nicotinic antagonists** bind nicotinic cholinoceptors in the muscle end-plate region.

    1. The **end-plate potential (EPP) is reduced** below the threshold for the muscle action potential.

    2. The **safety factor** is approximately **5** at the neuromuscular junction, thus the EPP must be reduced to 20% of the normal amplitude for muscle paralysis to occur.

        a. A **reduction of the safety factor** and an increase in the sensitivity to competitive neuromuscular blocking drugs occurs with:

            (1) **Myasthenia gravis**

            (2) **General anesthetics,** which reduce the sodium and potassium permeability changes at the end-plate.

            (3) **Aminoglycoside antibiotics,** which reduce the release of ACh.

        b. An **increase in the safety factor** and a reversal of competitive neuromuscular blockade can be induced with the **cholinesterase inhibitors** (e.g., neostigmine).

    3. All the competitive neuromuscular blocking drugs act by the same mechanism, but they do have other properties that are different.

        a. *d*-Tubocurarine:

            (1) **Releases histamine,** which can lead to bronchospasm and lower blood pressure

            (2) **Blocks ganglionic nicotinic receptors,** which can also lower blood pressure

        b. **Pancuronium** (*Pavulon*) induces a vagal blockade which can increase heart rate and increase blood pressure.

        c. **Atracurium** (*Tracrium*) is very short acting.

        d. **Vecuronium** (*Norcuron*) has no cardiovascular side effects.

C. **Depolarizing** neuromuscular blocking drugs act like ACh. **Succinylcholine** (*Anectine*) is a quaternary amine.

    1. It binds to and **activates the nicotinic cholinoceptors.**

        a. The **events, leading to Phase 1 depolarization block,** are **initiated** (Figure 2–8).

        b. With long periods of paralysis, Phase 2 block characterized by receptor desensitization develops.

    2. Succinylcholine is **metabolized by butyrylcholinesterases** in the serum.

        a. **Succinylcholine apnea** can occur if a patient has a **genetic** defect that results in low butyrylcholinesterase activity.

            (1) **Excessive paralysis will be induced by a standard dose,** because less of the drug is metabolized before reaching the end-plate region.

            (2) **Paralysis of the respiratory muscles** (apnea) occurs with an over-dose.

        b. There is **no antidote** for succinylcholine paralysis.

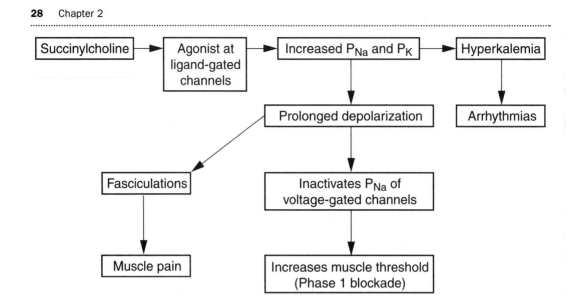

Figure 2-8. Effects of depolarizing neuromuscular blocking drugs (e.g., succinylcholine). P_{Na}= sodium permeability. P_K=potassium permeability

(1) Cholinesterase inhibitors will increase the paralysis by slowing the breakdown of succinylcholine and ACh.

(2) Patients should be **ventilated** until the respiratory function returns.

3. The major advantage of succinylcholine is the **rapid onset and short duration** of paralysis.

D. The primary **uses** of neuromuscular blocking drugs are as an adjunct during **intubation** and for **muscle relaxation during surgery.**

E. Other drugs can affect muscle function by various mechanisms.

1. **Hemicholinium** blocks the uptake of choline and leads to a depletion of ACh in the motor nerve terminal.

2. **Botulinum toxin** blocks the release of ACh which induces a muscle paralysis.

3. **α-Bungarotoxin** binds irreversibly to the neuromuscular nicotinic cholinoceptor.

4. **Dantrolene** (*Dantrium*) reduces calcium release from the sarcoplasmic reticulum in skeletal muscle. This reduces the spasticity from **malignant hyperthermia** (e.g., as induced by inhalation anesthetics and neuromuscular blocking drugs).

5. **Baclofen** (*Lioresal*) is a central muscle relaxant that activates $GABA_B$ receptors and thereby decreases spasticity.

XII. DRUGS FOR GASTROINTESTINAL DISORDERS

A. Ulcers can be treated in many ways.

1. **Triple antibiotic therapy** (e.g., bismuth salts, tetracyclines, and metronidazole) will kill the *Helicobacter pylori* that causes the ulcers.

   a. A permanent **cure** can be produced in many patients.

b. Antibiotic therapy is **inappropriate for salicylate-induced and nonsteroidal anti-inflammatory drug (NSAID)-induced ulcers.**

2. H$_2$-Antihistamines, such as cimetidine (*Tagamet*) and ranitidine (*Zantac*), are competitive antagonists at H$_2$-receptors in the intestinal tract.
   a. **Acid and pepsin secretion** are **reduced.**
   b. The release of intrinsic factor is unchanged.
   c. There are **no effects at H$_1$-receptors.**
   d. **Side effects** can occur.
      (1) **Cimetidine:**
         (a) Can cause **impotence** and **swelling of the breasts** due to antiandrogen activity.
         (b) **Increases prolactin release,** which can cause galactorrhea
         (c) **Inhibits mixed function oxidases,** which can slow the metabolism of many drugs (e.g., warfarin, propranolol) and enhance their effects.
      (2) Ranitidine has **fewer side effects** and a **longer duration** of action.

3. Sucralfate (*Carafate*) adheres to the ulcerated mucosal wall of the stomach and provides a **barrier** to acid and pepsin.

4. Omeprazole (*Prilosec*) **induces an irreversible inhibition of H$^+$/K$^+$ ATPase.**
   a. Acid secretion is decreased.
   b. It is very effective, especially for gastroesophageal reflux (heartburn).

5. Antacids directly neutralize stomach acid, however their duration of action is limited by the stomach emptying time.
   a. **Sodium bicarbonate** is a **systemic** antacid.
      (1) It is readily absorbed into the body.
      (2) **Side effects** are common, including:
         (a) **Metabolic alkalosis**
         (b) **Hypernatremia**
         (c) **Fluid retention**
         (d) **Acid rebound,** due to high gastric pH
   b. **Non-systemic** antacids are poorly absorbed into the body.
      (1) **Magnesium hydroxide** induces the side effect of **diarrhea.**
      (2) **Aluminum hydroxide** induces **constipation.**
      (3) Magnesium hydroxide and aluminum hydroxide are frequently combined to create an antacid preparation with little effect on GI motility.
      (4) **Calcium carbonate** (*Tums*) has more **side effects,** including:
         (a) **Hypercalcemia** (e.g., milk alkali syndrome)
         (b) **Acid rebound**
         (c) **Constipation**

6. Metoclopramide (*Octamide,Reglan*) and **cisapride** (*Propulsid*) are **cholinomimetics** that **increase lower esophageal sphincter tone.**
   a. Gastroesophageal reflux is decreased.
   b. Metoclopramide also has anti-emetic actions.

7. **Misoprostol** (*Cytotec*), a prostaglandin analogue, enhances the mucosal barrier and is used for **NSAID-induced** ulcers.

B. **Antidiarrheal drugs** are useful to reduce the loss of fluid and electrolytes that occurs with diarrhea. These drugs **should not be used for treating diarrhea that is caused by a poison, an infection, or chronic ulcerative colitis.**

1. **Opiates** act by increasing the tone and reducing the motility of the GI tract.
   a. **Diphenoxylate,** which is insoluble and poorly absorbed, is combined **with atropine** (*Lomotil*).
   b. **Loperamide** (*Imodium*) has no systemic side effects.

2. **Antimuscarinics** are ineffective for diarrhea, but will reduce the cramping from irritable bowel syndrome.

3. **Attapulgite,** a hydrophilic substance, absorbs water and reduces the looseness of the feces.

C. **Laxative-cathartics** add bulk and water to the feces, thereby stimulating peristalsis and relieving constipation. They should **never be used for undiagnosed abdominal pain or when intestinal obstruction is possible.**

   1. **Bulk laxatives** (e.g., psyllium and methylcellulose) are **fiber,** which increases the volume of the GI contents.

   2. **Docusate** (*Colace, Doxinate*) is a **fecal softener** that makes the passage of stools easier.

   3. **Castor oil** and **phenolphthalein** are contact laxatives.
      a. The active metabolite of castor oil is ricinoleic acid.
      b. **Irritation of nerve endings** increases peristaltic contractions.
      c. Prolonged use can lead to irritable bowel syndrome.

   4. **Osmotic (bulk) cathartics** are also called saline laxatives.
      a. **Magnesium sulfate** causes osmotic retention of large amounts of water in the gut.
      b. The increased bulk **enhances peristalsis.**

3

Cardiovascular Pharmacology

I. DIURETICS

A. Drugs in this class act on the kidney to **enhance the elimination of salt and water** from the body.

B. Increased intake of water does increase urine volume, due to decreased antidiuretic hormone (ADH) and decreased renin. Water is not a diuretic, however, because there is no net loss of body fluids.

C. **Ammonium chloride** induces a transient diuresis, and is useful only for:

    1. **Acidifying the urine** and increasing the elimination of weak bases

    2. **Treating metabolic alkalosis**

D. **Osmotic diuretics** [e.g., mannitol (*Osmitrol*), glycerol, urea] are **filtered by the kidney and not reabsorbed;** thus, these diuretics osmotically hold water in the tubules and increase urine flow. They can, however, increase extracellular volume, resulting in edema.

E. The **xanthines** (e.g., caffeine, theophylline, theobromine) produce a weak diuresis by increasing the glomerular filtration rate.

F. **Carbonic anhydrase inhibitors** [e.g., acetazolamide (*Diamox*)] **induce a bicarbonate loss** which leads to an alkaline diuresis.

G. **Thiazide** [e.g., hydrochlorothiazide (*Esidrix,HydroDIURIL*)] and thiazide-like [e.g. chlorthalidone (*Hygroton,Thalitone*)] diuretics act by **impairing the sodium and chloride cotransport** in the **initial part of the distal tubule.**

    1. The increased sodium in the tubular fluid holds water in the nephron, leading to the diuresis.

    2. The increased sodium in the tubular fluid also enhances Na^+/K^+ exchange, leading to a **hypokalemia.**

    3. The thiazides are effective when taken orally and are **eliminated by active proximal tubular secretion.**
        a. The secretion is important for the drugs to reach their intra-tubular site of action.
        b. Competition with the transport of uric acid at the same site can lead to hyperuricemia.

    4. Side effects from the thiazides include:
        a. **Hypokalemia,** which can increase the toxicity of the **cardiac glycosides**
        b. **Hyperuricemia**

    c. Hyperglycemia

    d. Small increases in low density lipoprotein (LDL) cholesterol

    e. Hypercalcemia

H. **Potassium-sparing diuretics** induce a weak diuresis by **reducing the sodium–potassium exchange** in the **late portion of the distal tubule and collecting ducts.** The serum potassium is also elevated as a result of this action.

  1. **Spironolactone** (*Aldactone*) is a **competitive aldosterone antagonist,** and it acts only when aldosterone is present.

  2. **Triamterene** (*Dyrenium*) and **amiloride** (*Midamor*) act directly on the sodium–potassium transport process and are effective even after an adrenalectomy and loss of endogenous aldosterone.

  3. These drugs cause:

    a. Potassium retention

    b. Small sodium loss

    c. Weak diuresis

  4. Side effects:

    a. Hyperkalemia

      (1) The potassium-sparing diuretics are frequently combined with thiazide and loop diuretics to counteract the hypokalemia from those diuretics.

      (2) If the acute risk of cardiac arrhythmias from the hyperkalemia is high, administration of insulin will reduce the hyperkalemia by enhancing potassium uptake into cells.

    b. **Gynecomastia** can be induced by spironolactone, which is a steroid antagonist.

    c. **Menstrual irregularities** can also result from the use of spironolactone.

I. The **loop diuretics** [furosemide (*Lasix*), ethacrynic acid (*Edecrin*) and bumetanide (*Bumex*)] are so named because they act at the **thick, ascending limb of the loop of Henle.**

  1. **Sodium and chloride cotransport is blocked.**

  2. **A marked diuresis is produced,** because large amounts of sodium are reabsorbed at this site.

  3. They are effective when taken orally and are **eliminated by active proximal tubular secretion.**

    a. The secretion is important for the drugs to reach their intra-tubular site of action.

    b. Competition with the transport of uric acid at the same site can lead to hyperuricemia.

    c. They have much shorter durations of action than the thiazides.

  4. Side effects are more common than with the thiazides and include:

    a. Hypovolemia

    b. Hyponatremia

    c. Hypokalemia, which increases the toxicity of the cardiac glycosides

    d. Hyperuricemia

    e. Hyperglycemia

    f. Hypocalcemia, which is the opposite of the effect of the thiazides

    g. Ototoxicity, especially with ethacrynic acid. Loop diuretics should not be combined with other ototoxic drugs (e.g., aminoglycosides).

  5. The loop diuretics have a **greater diuretic efficacy than the thiazides, which have a greater efficacy than the potassium-sparing diuretics.**

J. The diuretics are useful to **mobilize edematous fluid** from many sites in the body. Important **clinical indications for administration of diuretics** include:

1. **Congestive heart failure**—the diuretics will reduce the preload on the heart and improve heart function

2. **Hypertension**

3. **Hepatic ascites**

4. **Acute pulmonary edema**

5. **Renal failure**

6. **Hypercalcemia**—can be treated with furosemide

7. **Hypocalcemia**—can be treated with a thiazide

8. **Nephrogenic diabetes insipidus**—can be treated with a thiazide

9. **Inappropriate ADH secretion**—can be treated with furosemide and hypertonic saline

10. **Increased intracranial pressure**—can be treated with an osmotic agent

11. **Hyperaldosteronism**—can be treated with spironolactone

II. ANGIOTENSIN II AND ANGIOTENSIN BLOCKERS

A. The **synthesis** of angiotensin II and III are illustrated in Figure 3–1.

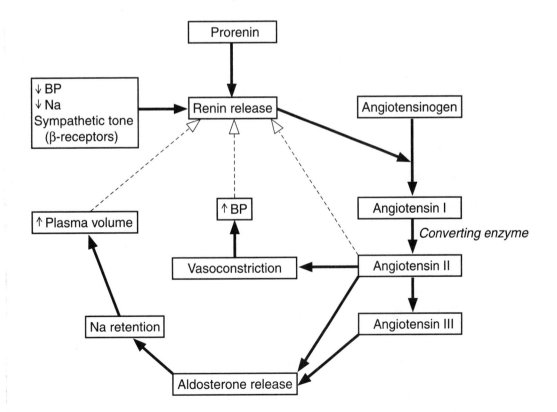

Figure 3-1. Renin-angiotensin system

B. Effects of angiotensin II include:

1. Vasoconstriction

2. Increased aldosterone release

3. Reduced renin release

C. The primary clinical **use** of angiotensin is to **increase blood pressure.** It induces fewer cardiac arrhythmias than the catecholamines.

D. **Angiotensin converting enzyme (ACE) can be inhibited** by several drugs.

1. **Captopril** (*Capoten*) is an ACE inhibitor.
   a. The **effects** of ACE inhibition include:
      (1) **Reduced conversion of angiotensin I to angiotensin II**
      (2) **Reduced blood pressure**
      (3) **Reduced aldosterone levels,** which increases sodium excretion
      (4) **Increased plasma renin levels,** due to reduced feedback inhibition on renin release
      (5) **Dilation of efferent renal arterioles,** which are regulated by angiotensin II.
   b. The **indications** for ACE inhibitors are:
      (1) **Hypertension**
      (2) **Congestive heart failure**
      (3) **Diabetic nephropathy**
   c. The **side effects** include:
      (1) **Hyperkalemia,** due to reduced aldosterone levels
      (2) **Hypotension**
      (3) **Coughing,** due to **increased bradykinin.** Converting enzyme also breaks down bradykinin.

2. **Enalapril** (*Vasotec*) and **lisinopril** (*Prinivil,Zestril*) have the same effects as captopril, but have **longer durations of action.**

E. The **AT1 angiotensin receptors can be inhibited by losartan** (*Cozaar*).

1. The effects are similar to those from ACE inhibitors.

2. **Coughing is less common** because converting enzyme is not inhibited.

III. BRADYKININ

A. Effects

1. A direct action on vascular smooth muscle leads to a **vasodilation.**

2. Stimulation of the sensory nerve endings induces **pain.**

3. Most non-vascular smooth muscle is contracted.

4. Capillary permeability is increased.

B. Bradykinin has no clinical usefulness.

IV. CALCIUM CHANNEL BLOCKERS

A. Drugs in this class **block the slow calcium channels,** especially the voltage-sensitive calcium channels. Calcium channel blockade primarily affects the cardiovascular system.

1. Reduced calcium entry **reduces the plateau phase** (phase 2) of the action potential in the sinoatrial (SA) and atrioventricular (AV) nodes of the heart. There is little effect on the ventricular action potential, where calcium currents are less important.

2. Reduced calcium entry into vascular smooth muscle leads to a **vasodilation** and fall in blood pressure.

B. Verapamil (*Calan,Isoptin*) and **diltiazem** (*Cardizem*):

1. Reduce heart rate

2. Prolong AV conduction time

3. Dilate coronary vessels

4. Dilate peripheral arterioles, without affecting venules

5. Reduce myocardial contractility

C. Nifedipine (*Procardia*) is a much **more potent arterial vasodilator** and the fall in blood pressure activates baroreceptor reflexes. As a result, the myocardial depressant effects from calcium channel blockade are counteracted, and:

1. Heart rate is increased

2. AV conduction time is reduced

3. Myocardial contractility is increased

D. Amlodipine (*Norvasc*) is a long-acting calcium channel blocker with properties similar to nifedipine.

E. The **clinical indications** for the calcium channel blockers are:

1. Supraventricular arrhythmias
  a. Paroxysmal supraventricular tachycardia (PSVT) can be acutely terminated.
  b. Atrial flutter and fibrillation are effectively treated, because reduced AV conduction due to the calcium channel blockade reduces the ventricular rate.

2. Angina

3. Hypertension

4. Cerebral vasospasm. Nimodipine (*Nimotop*) has a high lipid solubility and is particularly effective.

5. Vascular disease

6. Migraine headaches

V. ANTIHYPERTENSIVES

A. Treatment with antihypertensives is usually **initiated if the diastolic blood pressure is greater than 90–95 mm Hg.** Treatment has been demonstrated to **decrease the incidence of:**

1. Strokes

2. Heart failure

3. Myocardial infarctions

4. Coronary artery disease

5. Renal failure

B. **Treatment** is initiated with a **step one** drug.

1. Captopril (*Capoten*) inhibits ACE.
   a. This **reduces angiotensin synthesis** and **lowers blood pressure** by:
      (1) Vasodilating
      (2) **Reducing aldosterone release,** which increases the loss of water.
   b. There are no autonomic effects and no changes in LDL cholesterol, thus the **major side effects** are:
      (1) Hyperkalemia
      (2) Hypotension
   c. ACE inhibitors should be avoided in patients with renal artery stenosis because dilation of the efferent renal arterioles can excessively reduce the pressure in the glomerulus.

2. β-Blockers [e.g., propranolol (*Inderal*)] have many effects on blood pressure.
   a. The **mechanism** may be related to:
      (1) **Decreased heart rate and contractility**
      (2) **Decreased renin release**
      (3) **Decreased CNS sympathetic output**
      (4) **Blockade of presynaptic β-adrenoceptors** resulting in decreased norepinephrine (NE) release.
   b. The **side effects** are described in **Table 2–6.** Additional concerns are increased LDL cholesterol, increased triglycerides, and reduced high density lipoprotein (HDL) cholesterol.
   c. When combined with other antihypertensives, propranolol decreases the reflex sympathetic activation of the heart and the reflex sympathetic activation of renin release.
   d. **Metoprolol is cardioselective,** thus it induces less bronchoconstriction in asthmatics and less masking of hypoglycemia in diabetics than propranolol. The β-selectivity is relative, however, and tends to disappear at high dosages.

3. Thiazide diuretics [e.g., hydrochlorothiazide (*Esidrix, HydroDIURIL*)] **initially increase sodium and water loss.**
   a. This effect is compensated for by the mechanisms illustrated in Figure 3–2.
   b. **Later,** the blood pressure is reduced as a result of a **direct vasodilation** which decreases peripheral resistance.

Figure 3-2. Effects of the thiazides that reduce blood pressure and activate homeostatic mechanisms

    c. High salt intake leads to water retention which will reduce the effectiveness of the thiazides.

    d. The **onset of the antihypertensive action is slow,** taking 2–4 weeks to develop.

    e. **Side effects** can occur, including:

      (1) **Hypokalemia**

        (a) To avoid hypokalemia, combine thiazide diuretics with potassium supplements or potassium-sparing diuretics.

        (b) This is especially important for patients on cardiac glycosides.

      (2) **Hyperglycemia**

      (3) **Increased LDL and reduced HDL cholesterol**

    f. The loop diuretics should be used only if the thiazides do not induce a diuresis.

  4. **Calcium channel blockers** [e.g., amlodipine (*Norvasc*)] vasodilate arterioles and reduce blood pressure. They have no autonomic side effects and do not change the LDL cholesterol.

C. **Step two** drugs are the **sympathetic blockers,** which can be used alone, but are usually combined with a step one drug.

  1. **Prazosin** is an α_1-blocker.

  2. **Labetalol** is an α_1 and β-blocker.

  3. **Clonidine** decreases CNS sympathetic output.

  4. **Methyldopa** decreases CNS sympathetic output.

D. **Step three** drugs [e.g., hydralazine (*Apresoline*), minoxidil (*Loniten*)] are **arteriolar vasodilators.**

  1. A **direct** vasodilation of arterioles leads to a fall in blood pressure.

  2. **Homeostatic mechanisms** (e.g., sympathetic reflexes) are induced, which compensate for the fall in blood pressure and make the arteriolar vasodilators **ineffective when used alone.** The homeostatic mechanisms include:

    a. An increase in sympathetic vasoconstrictor tone to blood vessels

    b. An increase in heart rate

    c. An increase in myocardial contractility

    d. An increase in renin release

  3. The vasodilators are usually **combined with diuretics and sympathetic blockers,** which will dampen the homeostatic compensatory mechanisms.

  4. **Side effects** of these drugs include:

    a. **Palpitations**

    b. **Flushing**

    c. **Headache**

    d. **Lupus-like syndrome with hydralazine,** especially in patients who are slow acetylators.

    e. **Hirsutism with minoxidil.** In fact, minoxidil is used topically (as *Rogaine*) to treat baldness.

    f. **Pericardial effusion with minoxidil**

VI. DRUGS FOR HYPERTENSIVE CRISES

A. Hypertensive crisis may be caused by secondary mechanisms. If it is due to **elevated catecholamines,** a **phentolamine test** can be used for the diagnosis.

  1. Phentolamine will **rapidly reduce blood pressure that has been elevated** due to:

    a. Pheochromocytoma

    b. Monoamine oxidase inhibitors

    c. Sympathomimetics or cocaine

    d. Clonidine withdrawal

2. **Measurement of urinary catecholamine metabolites** is also diagnostic.

3. **Treatment of hypertensive crises due to elevated catecholamines** involves the administration of:

    a. **α- and β-blockers**

    b. Labetalol

    c. Metyrosine, an inhibitor of tyrosine hydroxylase

B. **Hypertensive crises due to other causes** will not respond so dramatically to phentolamine and are treated with rapid-acting antihypertensives.

    1. **Sodium nitroprusside** (*Nipride*), like the nitrates, **dilates venules** and **arterioles.**

        a. The onset of action is **very rapid,** within minutes.

        b. The half-life is **very short,** which makes the antihypertensive effect **very controllable,** but it requires regular monitoring.

        c. **Side effects** include:

            (1) Hypotension

            (2) **Toxicity from thiocyanate and cyanide,** which are by-products of nitroprusside metabolism.

    2. **Diazoxide** (*Hyperstat I.V.*), like hydralazine, **dilates only arterioles.**

        a. **Side effects** include:

            (1) Palpitations

            (2) Hyperglycemia

        b. It can **aggravate angina.**

    3. **Trimethaphan** (*Arfonad*) is a rapid-acting **ganglionic blocker** that decreases sympathetic tone to the blood vessels.

    4. **Nifedipine** (*Procardia*), a **calcium channel blocker** that dilates arterioles, has a very rapid onset when administered sublingually.

    5. **Labetalol** (*Normodyne, Trandate*), when administered intravenously, has a rapid onset.

VII. DRUGS FOR ANGINA PECTORIS

A. Patients with angina (stable, variant, or unstable types) develop **S-T segment elevation or depression** on the electrocardiogram (EKG) during myocardial hypoxia. This can be induced diagnostically by:

    1. Treadmill stress testing

    2. Ergonovine, which induces a coronary vasoconstriction

    3. Dobutamine, which increases heart rate and contractility

B. **Treatment** is oriented to reducing oxygen demand or increasing oxygen supply to the heart.

    1. **Nitrates,** which are useful for all types of angina, act directly on vascular smooth muscle cells.

        a. They dilate vessels in a manner similar to nitric oxide. Endothelium-derived relaxing factor (EDRF) is probably nitric oxide.

            (1) The primary effect is a **reduction in venous tone,** which leads to venous pooling and reduced venous return (reduced preload).

(2) Arteriolar tone is less effectively reduced, and leads to reduced peripheral resistance (reduced afterload) and reduced blood pressure.

(3) Both effects reduce the myocardial wall stress and thereby **reduce the oxygen consumption** of the heart.

(4) Dilation of collateral coronary vessels and coronary vessels in spasm are additional minor effects.

b. Short and long acting **preparations** are available.

(1) **Nitroglycerin** (*Nitrostat*) is administered **sublingually** to terminate an acute anginal attack.

(a) The onset is very rapid and the half–life is short (1–3 minutes).

(b) Oral administration is ineffective for the treatment of an acute attack due to a high first–pass metabolism.

(2) High doses of nitroglycerin (*Nitro-Bid*), which saturate the metabolic enzymes, can be administered orally or topically for prophylaxis.

(3) **Isosorbide dinitrate** (*Isordil*) is a long-acting nitrate that is also useful for prophylaxis.

c. Side effects from the nitrates include:

(1) **Headache** from the vascular dilation

(2) **Syncope** from the **postural hypotension**

(3) **Reflex tachycardia,** which may occasionally induce an anginal attack

(4) **Methemoglobinemia,** which can be reversed by methylene blue

(5) **Tolerance and withdrawal symptoms,** such as anginal attacks during withdrawal from high-dose, long-term therapy

2. **β-Blockers** produce several beneficial effects.

a. β-Blockade of the heart is very important.

(1) Exercise-induced tachycardia and exercise-induced increases in myocardial contractility are reduced.

(2) Blood pressure is decreased (decreased afterload).

(3) Heart rate is reduced, which increases endocardial perfusion time.

(4) Reflex tachycardia from the nitrates is reduced, making the combination of nitrates and β-blockers quite useful.

b. **Propranolol should be avoided** or used with caution in patients with:

(1) **Congestive heart failure,** due to the depressant effect on myocardial contractility

(2) **Variant angina,** as blockade of β-adrenoceptors (dilatory) in the coronary vessels may increase the coronary spasm

(3) **Asthma,** due to a bronchoconstricting effect

(4) **Calcium channel blockers,** as both classes of drugs depress myocardial contractility

c. **Propranolol is used prophylactically for 1.5 to 3 years after an acute MI to decrease the ischemic damage.**

d. The side effects of β-blockers have been previously described (See Table 2–6). It is important to **avoid rapid withdrawal** from treatment, which can induce anginal attacks.

3. **Calcium channel blockers** [e.g., verapamil (*Calan, Isoptin*)] are effective for the treatment of all types of angina, and may be used in combination with the nitrates or the β-blockers or both. Calcium channel blockers

a. **Decrease heart rate**

b. **Decrease myocardial contractility**

c. **Vasodilate arterioles** (decrease afterload)

d. **Dilate coronary vessels,** which reduces coronary spasm

VIII. CARDIAC GLYCOSIDES

A. The cardiac glycosides are derived from the foxglove (*Digitalis*) plant.

B. These drugs **inhibit Na⁺/K⁺ ATPase,** which **reduces active Na⁺/K⁺ transport** and increases the intracellular concentrations of sodium and **calcium** ions. The elevated free calcium ion concentration enhances myocardial contractility.

   1. The effect on ventricular performance is shown in Figure 3–3.
      a. No net change of oxygen consumption occurs.
      b. The efficiency of myocardial contractions is improved.

   2. The increased contractility leads to a cascade of events shown in Figure 3–4.

C. Two glycosides are used clinically.

   1. Digoxin (*Lanoxin*) has a bioavailability of 75% and a volume of distribution (V_d) of 6 l/kg, due to accumulation in tissues, but not in fat. Generic preparations are not reliably bioequivalent.
      a. It is **eliminated primarily by glomerular filtration in the kidney,** thus the **creatinine clearance** is useful in determining the maintenance dose.

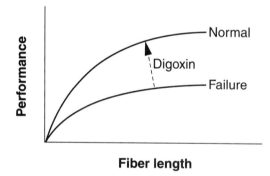

Figure 3-3.   Effect of digoxin on myocardial contractility.

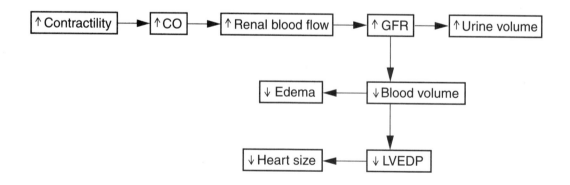

Figure 3-4.   Effects resulting from the increase in myocardial contractility induced by digoxin. CO=cardiac output; GFR=glomerular filtration rate; LVEDP=left ventricular end-diastolic pressure

  b. The **half-life is 36 hours,** which means that a steady state serum drug concentration is not achieved for 6–8 days (without a loading dose).

  c. For a rapid onset of action, use a divided loading dose to avoid toxicity.

 2. Digitoxin (*Crystodigin*) is more lipid soluble and has a bioavailability of 100%.

  a. It is 97% bound to plasma proteins.

  b. Digitoxin is **cleared by metabolism** in the liver and the metabolite is eliminated in the bile. 25% is reabsorbed (enterohepatic cycling).

  c. The **half-life is 5–7 days.**

D. The **indications** for the glycosides are:

 1. **Severe, chronic congestive heart failure** (but not high output, obstructive, or pulmonary failure)

  a. **ACE inhibitors** are preferred for the treatment of **mild congestive heart failure.**

  b. **Hypertrophic cardiomyopathy,** which can lead to heart failure, is best treated with β-blockers or **calcium channel blockers** to reduce heart rate and thereby enhance the filling of the heart.

 2. **Supraventricular arrhythmias** (e.g., atrial flutter and atrial fibrillation). The glycosides reduce the ventricular rate by inducing partial AV nodal block.

E. **Side effects** are very common, because there is considerable overlap between the therapeutic and toxic serum concentration ranges.

 1. **Cardiac toxicities** can be life-threatening.

  a. **Vagal enhancement** can lead to **bradycardia** and **AV nodal block** (indirect effects). These side effects can be treated with atropine.

  b. **Direct actions** on the myocardium (from ATPase inhibition) can lead to **arrhythmias** that are accentuated by hypokalemia (e.g., from diuretics). This side effect can be treated with potassium or lidocaine.

 2. Non-cardiac effects are usually not life-threatening.

  a. **Nausea and vomiting** occurs due to activation of the chemoreceptor trigger zone (CTZ) in the CNS.

  b. Enhanced vagal activity can lead to **diarrhea.**

  c. **Color vision** can be distorted.

F. If the toxicity is mild (and serum potassium is in the normal range), withdraw the glycoside and restart at a lower dose. If toxicity is life-threatening, administer digoxin immune F_{ab} (*Digibind*).

G. **Drug interactions** are common.

 1. **Hypokalemia** or **hypercalcemia** increase toxicity.

 2. Reduced renal clearance of digoxin, leading to increased toxicity, occurs with:

  a. Quinidine

  b. Calcium channel blockers

  c. Hypothyroidism

IX. ANTIARRHYTHMICS

A. There are 5 phases in the cardiac action potential:

 1. Phase 0—upstroke due to the sodium current

 2. Phase 1—peak

 3. Phase 2—plateau due to the calcium current

4. Phase 3—repolarization due to the potassium current

5. Phase 4—diastolic depolarization

B. **Bradyarrhythmias** can be treated with **atropine or β-agonists.**

C. **Tachyarrhythmias** can be treated with the **antiarrhythmics,** which depress the electrical activity of the myocardial cells. The antiarrhythmics reduce tachyarrhythmias by:

    1. Decreasing ectopic automaticity

    2. Increasing or decreasing conduction, to reduce reentry

D. There are **4 mechanisms** of **antiarrhythmic action,** including:

    1. Sodium channel blockade

    2. β-Blockade

    3. Increased refractoriness

    4. Calcium channel blockade

E. **Class IA** antiarrhythmics are **sodium channel blockers** (direct action) with anticholinergic activity (indirect action).

    1. The **effects** of the two actions are illustrated in **Table 3–1.**

    2. The changes of the myocardial action potential are illustrated in Figure 3–5.
        a. The **slowing of the diastolic depolarization** (Phase 4) leads to the reduced automaticity.
        b. The **slowing of the rate of rise** of the action potential (Phase O) leads to the reduced excitability and reduced conduction velocity.
        c. The **prolongation** of the action potential leads to the increased effective refractory period.

    3. The **indirect actions** from the **anticholinergic activity** only occur at the SA and AV nodes because these are the primary sites of parasympathetic innervation.
        a. The net effect of the IA antiarrhythmics at the SA and AV nodes is variable, depending upon whether the direct or indirect effects predominate.
        b. At atrial and ventricular muscle, the direct effects predominate, because there is little parasympathetic innervation.

    4. Class IA antiarrhythmics are **often combined with the cardiac glycosides.**

Table 3-1
Changes in Myocardial Cell Properties due to the Direct (Sodium Channel Block) and Indirect (Vagal Block) Actions of the Group IA Antiarrhythmics

Sodium channel block	Vagal block (SA and AV nodes)
↓ automaticity	↑ automaticity
↓ excitability	↑ excitability
↑ effective refractory period	↓ effective refractory period
Sum total of effects of IA antiarrhythmics: at SA and AV nodes—variable effects at atrial and ventricular muscle—direct effects	

AV=atrioventricular; SA=sinoatrial; ↑=increased; ↓=decreased

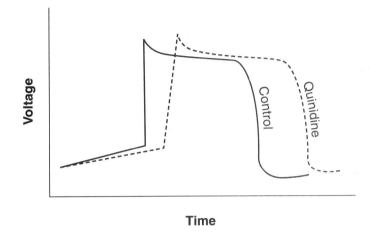

Figure 3-5. Changes in the myocardial action potential induced by Class IA antiarrhythmics (e.g., quinidine)

    a. The indirect effects (anticholinergic) of the antiarrhythmic oppose the indirect effects (vagomimetic) of the cardiac glycoside.
    b. The combination results in little indirect activity, and leads to sodium channel blockade with increased myocardial contractility.

5. Several Class IA antiarrhythmics are commonly used.
    a. **Quinidine** (*Quinidex,Cardioquin*) is only used orally, as parenteral administration has marked hypotensive effects.
        (1) The side effects include **cinchonism,** which is characterized by ringing in the ears, blurred vision, nausea, and vomiting.
        (2) Quinidine reduces the renal elimination of digoxin, which can lead to an increase in the toxicity from digoxin.
    b. **Procainamide** (*Pronestyl*) can be used orally or intravenously.
        (1) N-Acetylprocainamide is an active metabolite.
        (2) **A lupus-like syndrome** can be induced, especially in those patients who have a **slow acetylator phenotype.**
    c. **Disopyramide** (*Norpace*) is an oral antiarrhythmic that is also the most potent antimuscarinic.

6. Some **side effects** are common to all Class IA antiarrhythmics.
    a. **Ventricular arrhythmias** induced by the Class IA antiarrhythmics can lead to **syncope.**
    b. **AV block** induced by the Class IA antiarrhythmics can lead to an **increased P-R interval.**
    c. There may also be increased QRS and QT intervals.
    d. **Decreased contractility** can aggravate heart failure, especially with disopyramide.
    e. A direct **vasodilation** can lower blood pressure.

7. **Uses** for Class IA antiarrhythmic drugs are:

    a. Treatment and prophylactic control of symptomatic ventricular tachy-arrhythmias

    b. Prophylactic control of supraventricular arrhythmias.

F. **Class IB** antiarrhythmic drugs are **sodium channel blockers** without anticholinergic activity.

    1. Lidocaine (*Xylocaine*) is a very effective **parenteral** antiarrhythmic.

        a. It is rapidly metabolized in the liver **(high extraction ratio)** and has a low bioavailability (0.3); thus it is not used orally.

            (1) **Heart failure** will decrease the liver blood flow and thereby slow the metabolism of lidocaine.

            (2) The **maintenance dose** of lidocaine should be **reduced** in patients with heart failure.

        b. The **elimination of lidocaine** follows **2 compartment** kinetics (Figure 3–6), thus repeated dosing will increase the duration of the therapeutic effect.

        c. The **effects** of lidocaine **on the myocardial action potential** are illustrated in **Figure 3–7.**

            (1) **Automaticity is decreased.**

            (2) **Excitability is decreased.**

            (3) **The effective refractory period is decreased,** which is unexpected.

        d. The actions of lidocaine on myocardial muscle are **frequency-dependent,** with the highest activity at the higher frequencies. Thus it acts preferentially on arrhythmic muscle.

        e. There are **few side effects,** however **at large dosages** it can:

            (1) Produce local anesthetic side effects, such as **tremors** and **convulsions**

            (2) **Reduce myocardial contractility**

            (3) **Slow AV conduction**

        f. The **indications** for the use of lidocaine are limited to **ventricular** tachy-arrhythmias, including:

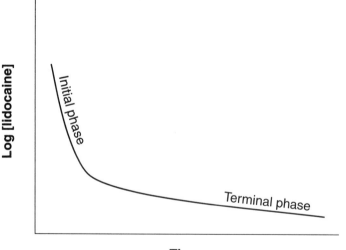

Figure 3-6.   Lidocaine concentration versus time relationship, which displays two phases (two compartments)

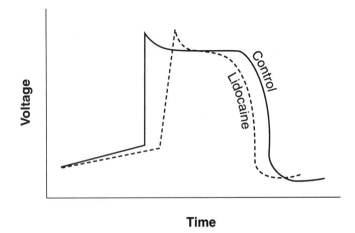

Figure 3-7. Changes in the myocardial action potential induced by Class IB antiarrhythmics (e.g., lidocaine)

    (1) Ventricular tachycardia
    (2) Premature ventricular complexes
    (3) Ventricular fibrillation
    (4) Digitalis-induced ventricular arrhythmias

  2. **Mexiletine** (*Mexitil*) has effects that are similar to lidocaine, and:
    a. It is **effective when given orally,** as there is no first–pass metabolism.
    b. The half-life is much **longer.**

  3. **Phenytoin** (*Dilantin*), an anticonvulsant, also has antiarrhythmic effects.

G. **Class IC** antiarrhythmic drugs [e.g., **flecainide** (*Tambocor*)] induce marked reductions of the sodium permeability changes.

H. **Class II** antiarrhythmics are the **β-blockers** [e.g., propranolol (*Inderal*)].

  1. They act primarily by **reducing the effects of the sympathetic nervous system on the myocardium.**
    a. **Phase 4 depolarization is reduced,** leading to a reduction of automaticity in the SA node, AV node and Purkinje fibers.
    b. **Excitability is reduced.**
    c. The effective refractory period of the AV node is increased.

  2. High doses may induce sodium channel blockade.

  3. Indications for β-blockers include:
    a. **Sympathetic-induced tachyarrhythmias**
    b. **PSVT** (because β-blockers reduce reentry at the AV node)
    c. **Atrial flutter and fibrillation** (because β-blockers slow AV conduction, thereby reducing the ventricular rate)
    d. **Prophylaxis after an acute MI** (because β-blockers reduce sudden death)

I. Class III antiarrhythmics **prolong the action potential and the effective refractory period.**

    1. Amiodarone (*Cordarone*) increases the refractory period.

        a. It **acts at all sites** in the myocardium, which is unusual for an antiarrhythmic, and it effectively reduces almost any arrhythmia.

        b. The **half-life is very long,** approximately 30 days.

        c. **Toxicity is very high,** including:

            (1) **Pneumonitis.** Pulmonary toxicity is fatal in 10% of patients affected.

            (2) Change of thyroid function

    2. Bretylium (*Bretylol*) decreases catecholamine release, prolongs the action potential, and increases the effective refractory period in the myocardium.

    3. Sotalol (*Betapace*) is a non-selective β-blocker with Class III activity.

J. Class IV antiarrhythmics are the **calcium channel blockers** [e.g., **verapamil** (*Calan, Isoptin*)].

    1. Calcium channels are particularly important for action potential generation in the SA and AV nodes.

    2. Blockade of the calcium channels **decreases heart rate, slows AV conduction,** and **increases the effective refractory period.**

    3. Verapamil has a low bioavailability (F = 0.2), due to first-pass metabolism, and 80%–90% of the verapamil in the serum is bound to plasma proteins.

    4. **Indications** for the calcium channel blockers include supraventricular arrhythmias, such as:

        a. **PSVT**

        b. **Atrial flutter**

        c. **Atrial fibrillation**

    5. **Side effects** of verapamil include:

        a. **Bradycardia**

        b. **AV block**

        c. **Heart failure,** due to reduced myocardial contractility

        d. Constipation

    6. The effects of the calcium channel blockers on the myocardium can be antagonized by the catecholamines, digoxin, or calcium.

K. **Miscellaneous** antiarrhythmics are also useful.

    1. **Adenosine** (*Adenocard*) hyperpolarizes supraventricular muscle membranes, and it is used to **terminate PSVT.** The duration of action is only one minute.

    2. **Digoxin** (*Lanoxin*) has antiarrhythmic effects, due to a **depression of AV nodal conduction.**

        a. Increased myocardial contractility and the long duration of action of digoxin are unusual for antiarrhythmics.

        b. Uses include:

            (1) **Atrial flutter and fibrillation**

            (2) **PSVT**

            (3) **Arrhythmias in patients with congestive heart failure**

    3. **Phenylephrine** increases blood pressure, which reflexly reduces heart rate and reduces PSVT.

    4. **Edrophonium** enhances vagal tone to the heart, which reduces heart rate and reduces PSVT.

X. ANTICOAGULANTS

A. Heparin (*Liquaemin*) is an **acidic mucopolysaccharide.**

1. High endogenous concentrations occur in the mast cells in the lungs.

2. It is a **very large, polar,** and **water-soluble molecule.**
   a. It must be **given intravenously** or **subcutaneously.**
   b. Distribution is limited to the **vascular space.**
   c. **Inactivation** is due to **metabolism,** which follows **zero–order kinetics.** Increasing the dose increases the time to eliminate 50% of the drug.

3. It acts by **catalyzing** the reaction between **antithrombin III** and **thrombin,** which results in an inactive complex of thrombin.
   a. It also **complexes factor Xa.**
   b. The onset of action is **immediate.**
   c. The goal of treatment is to increase the **activated partial thromboplastin time (APTT)** by approximately **2 times** the normal value.

4. **Side effects** include:
   a. **Hemorrhage**
   b. **Thrombocytopenia,** which is immunologically mediated.

5. **Protamine,** a basic compound which **complexes heparin,** is the **antidote** for heparin.

6. Low molecular weight heparins:
   a. **Act only on factor Xa.** Monitor the Xa concentration rather than APTT.
   b. Are better absorbed after subcutaneous injection than heparin
   c. Are eliminated by the kidney, by **first order kinetics.** They should not be used in patients with renal failure.
   d. Have a more predictable dose-response relationship than heparin
   e. Have a lower incidence of thrombocytopenia than heparin

B. Warfarin (*Coumadin,Panwarfin*) is an **oral anticoagulant.**

1. Blockade of the reduction of vitamin K to its active form slows the carboxylation and **decreases the synthesis of vitamin K-dependent clotting factors** (II, VII, IX and X).
   a. The **onset of action is delayed** (8–12 hours), because stores of the clotting factors must be depleted.
   b. The maximum anticoagulant effect of warfarin occurs after 1 week of administration.
   c. The therapeutic goal is to approximately double the prothrombin time.

2. Because warfarin is **effective when given orally,** it is more useful than heparin for outpatients.

3. **Many drug interactions** can occur.
   a. Extensive plasma protein binding (99%) can result in competition with other drugs for the binding sites.
   b. Metabolism of warfarin in the liver can be enhanced by many other drugs.

4. The **side effects include:**
   a. **Hemorrhage,** which can be reversed by the **antidotes, vitamin K or vitamin-K dependent clotting factors.**
   b. **Skin necrosis,** due to thrombosis of the microvasculature in the skin.
   c. **Teratogenicity,** because it readily crosses the placenta and affects the developing fetus.

5. Acute anticoagulant therapy is often initiated with both heparin and warfarin. As the warfarin becomes effective, the heparin is withdrawn.

6. Warfarin and heparin slow the production of a clot, but they do not dissolve clots.

C. Fibrinolytics dissolve clots.

1. Tissue plasminogen activator (tPA), urokinase, streptokinase and **anistreplase** enhance the formation of plasmin from plasminogen.
  a. The plasmin breaks down fibrin, thereby dissolving clots.
  b. Dissolution of clots by **intracoronary administration of a fibrinolytic** can restore coronary blood flow after an **MI.**
    (1) This will reduce myocardial damage, if given within a few hours of the MI.
    (2) It can also induce hemorrhaging at other sites.
  c. Dissolution of clots in the brain by fibrinolytics can reduce the CNS injury after a **thrombotic stroke.** It must not be used after a hemorrhagic stroke.

2. The **antidote** for the fibrinolytics is **aminocaproic acid,** a plasmin antagonist.

D. Antiplatelet drugs, given prophylactically, reduce the incidence of MI and stroke.

1. Low doses of aspirin inhibit cyclooxygenase which **decreases thromboxane synthesis,** thereby decreasing platelet aggregation.

2. Dipyridamole (*Persantine*) decreases platelet adhesiveness.

XI. DRUGS FOR SHOCK

A. The treatment for each type of shock will be quite different.

B. Avoid vasoconstrictors if the sympathetic nervous system has already compromised blood flow to the peripheral tissues.

C. Use fluids, vasodilators, and inotropic drugs. Dopamine is particularly useful because it will dilate the renal and mesenteric vasculature.

XII. ANTIHYPERLIPIDEMICS

A. The first mode of therapy for hypercholesterolemias is **modification of the diet** to reduce fat and caloric intake.

B. Lovastatin (*Mevacor*) and **simvastatin** (*Zocor*) **competitively inhibit hydroxymethylglutarylCoA (HMG CoA) reductase.**

1. This enzyme is the **rate limiting** step in the synthesis of cholesterol.

2. Reduced cholesterol synthesis leads to an increase in the number of hepatic **LDL receptors,** which then enhances the uptake of LDL cholesterol from the serum.
  a. Serum LDL cholesterol is reduced.
  b. HDL cholesterol is slightly increased.
  c. Triglycerides are slightly reduced.
  d. The risk of MI is reduced.

3. Side effects from lovastatin include
  a. Hepatotoxicity
  b. Myositis, an inflammation of skeletal muscle.

C. Cholestyramine (*Questran*) and **colestipol** (*Colestid*) are **quaternary ammonium ion-exchange resins** that are **not absorbed** from the intestine.

   1. They **bind bile salts** and eliminate them in the feces.
      a. Bile salt synthesis from cholesterol is increased.
      b. Cholesterol content in the liver is reduced.
      c. The liver increases the number of LDL receptors, which lowers the serum LDL cholesterol.

   2. Side effects include:
      a. Abdominal discomfort and constipation.
      b. Binding of fat-soluble vitamins and anionic drugs
      c. An increase in very low density lipoproteins (VLDL) and triglycerides.

D. Niacin (nicotinic acid, vitamin B_3) at high dosages has antihyperlipidemic actions.

   1. Many effects occur and the exact mechanism is unclear.
      a. It decreases lipolysis in adipose tissue which decreases the free fatty acids in the plasma.
      b. Triglyceride synthesis is reduced, which decreases the hepatic secretion of VLDL.
      c. Decreased LDL production leads to reduced serum cholesterol.

   2. A common **side effect** is **cutaneous flushing,** due to **prostaglandin** release. This effect can be reduced with **aspirin.**

E. **Gemfibrozil** (*Lopid*) and **clofibrate** (*Atromid-S*) are more active in **lowering triglycerides.**

   1. **Increases in lipoprotein lipase activity** lead to a reduction of VLDL, which predominantly transports triglycerides.

   2. Elimination of cholesterol in the bile is also enhanced and **gallstones** are a **side effect.**

4

Central Neuropharmacology

I. PRINCIPLES OF GENERAL ANESTHESIA

A. **The primary objectives** of general anesthesia are:

1. Amnesia

2. Analgesia

3. Blunting of consciousness

4. Suppression of autonomic reflexes

5. Muscle relaxation

B. Due to the blood-brain barrier, all central nervous system (CNS) drugs including the general anesthetics must either have some **lipid solubility** or be carried across the barrier by active transport in order to be effective.

C. The mechanism of action of general anesthetics involves a **physical association** with cell membranes. This leads to several implications.

1. The **potency** of each gaseous anesthetic, characterized by the **minimal anesthetic concentration (MAC),** is directly related to the **oil-water partition coefficient** for that anesthetic.

2. The association of the anesthetic with cell membranes **reduces the excitability** of the membranes.

3. There are **no receptors** for the anesthetics.

4. There are **no specific antagonists** for the anesthetics.

D. At low concentrations of a general anesthetic the CNS is depressed more than other tissues; but as the concentration is increased, all excitable cells are eventually depressed.

E. Anesthetics induce characteristic stages of anesthesia. These were first described for anesthesia with diethyl ether, but occur with other anesthetics as well.

1. Stage 1 involves **analgesia.**

2. Stage 2 involves **excitement,** due to **blockade of inhibitory pathways** in the brain. This can be a dangerous phase, due to the vomiting, restlessness, and other hyperexcitable effects that may occur.

3. Stage 3 is the stage at which **surgery is usually performed,** and Stage 3 is divided into four planes.

4. Stage 4 involves **respiratory and cardiovascular depression,** which, if pronounced, can lead to death.

F. The inhalation anesthetics act as gases in the body and follow the **gas laws.**

  1. Dalton's Law. An anesthetic exerts a partial pressure that is proportional to the percent of the anesthetic in the mixture.

  2. Fick's Law. The anesthetic diffuses down its concentration gradient.

  3. Henry's Law. The amount of anesthetic dissolved in a liquid is proportional to the partial pressure of the anesthetic in the mixture.

G. The **rate of induction** of anesthesia is **dependent on the blood solubility of an anesthetic.**

  1. The blood solubility can be determined by measuring the blood–gas partition coefficient (λ).

  2. High blood solubility leads to a slow rise in the partial pressure of the anesthetic in the body and a slow induction.

  3. The induction of highly blood soluble anesthetics is most readily hastened by hyperventilation.

H. The factors affecting distribution vary with the phase.

  1. The **initial distribution** of an anesthetic will be dependent on the relative **tissue blood flows,** going to areas with the higher blood flows.

  2. The **final distribution** will be dependent on the **tissue-blood partition coefficients,** although the tissue-blood partition coefficients for most anesthetics in most tissues is approximately one.
    a. An exception is the fat-blood partition coefficient which can be high for some anesthetics (e.g., halothane).
    b. Movement of halothane into fat will be slow due to the low blood supply to fat. Only after long anesthesias will significant amounts of halothane be sequestered in fat.
    c. Recovery from long anesthesias with halothane may be slower than normal due to the slow elimination of halothane from fat.

II. INHALATION ANESTHETICS

A. Diethyl ether was the first useful general anesthetic.

  1. It has several major **disadvantages,** including:
    a. Very slow induction ($\lambda = 16$)
    b. Flammability
    c. Respiratory irritation

  2. It is, however, a **complete anesthetic,** meaning that it induces:
    a. Muscle relaxation, due to actions on the spinal cord and neuromuscular junction
    b. Analgesia
    c. Unconsciousness

  3. In addition, it **maintains respiration and circulation.**

B. Most of the **newer anesthetics:**

  1. Have faster rates of induction and recovery, due to lower blood solubilities

  2. Are **non-flammable**

  3. Are **not irritating** to the respiratory tract

    4. Are **uterine relaxants**

    5. Are usually combined with other drugs (e.g., analgesics and muscle relaxants) to overcome their inherent disadvantages. The combination is called **balanced anesthesia.**

C. **Halothane** (*Fluothane*) with a λ of 2.3 was the first useful **halogenated hydrocarbon** anesthetic. It does have some disadvantages, however, in that it:

    1. Is a poor skeletal muscle relaxant

    2. Is a poor analgesic

    3. Is a strong respiratory depressant

    4. Is a strong cardiovascular depressant

    5. Is **metabolized** (approximately 20%) in the liver to halogenated products that appear to be **hepatotoxic**

    6. **Sensitizes the myocardium to catecholamines,** leading to arrhythmias when catecholamines are injected.

D. **Enflurane** (*Ethrane*) with a λ of 1.8 has many properties that are intermediate between halothane and diethyl ether. It:

    1. Induces some skeletal muscle relaxation

    2. Has some analgesic activity

    3. Is somewhat metabolized (approximately 2%)

    4. Induces some sensitization of the myocardium to catecholamines

    5. Can induce **seizure patterns** during anesthesia

E. **Isoflurane** (*Forane*) with a λ of 1.4 has:

    1. Some respiratory irritation

    2. Good skeletal muscle relaxation

    3. Good analgesia

    4. Low myocardial depression

    5. Fewer metabolites than enflurane

F. **Nitrous oxide** is a gas with:

    1. **A rapid onset and recovery** (λ = 0.4)

    2. **Excellent analgesic activity**

    3. No effect on the function of most vital systems

    4. **Inadequate potency,** leading to:
        a. Unconsciousness only when used with other anesthetics
        b. **A second gas effect** during induction which accelerates the onset of anesthesia by other inhalation anesthetics
        c. **Diffusion hypoxia** during recovery, due to the filling of the lungs with nitrous oxide so that inadequate oxygen is inhaled. This can be avoided by administering **100% oxygen** for a short time at the conclusion of the nitrous oxide anesthesia.

G. Several **miscellaneous** anesthetics are of historical interest.

    1. Methoxyflurane is:
      a. **The most potent anesthetic** available for clinical use
      b. **The best analgesic** anesthetic
      c. **Nephrotoxic** and thus seldom used

    2. **Cyclopropane** is an explosive gas.

    3. **Chloroform** is:
      a. A complete anesthetic
      b. Hepatotoxic

III. INTRAVENOUS ANESTHETICS

  A. Barbiturates

    1. **Thiopental** (*Pentothal*) has a rapid onset of anesthesia due to a **high lipid solubility.** When administered it goes primarily to areas of high blood flow, such as the brain.

    2. The short duration of anesthesia is due to **redistribution** from the brain to peripheral tissues with lower blood flows, such as skeletal muscle.

    3. Clearance from the body by metabolism is very slow.

    4. The duration of anesthesia becomes longer with repeated administrations because less redistribution can occur. As a result, the primary **uses** of thiopental are for:
      a. **Induction** of anesthesia
      b. **Short anesthesias**

    5. The anesthetic has the following **properties:**
      a. **Marked respiratory and cardiovascular depression,** especially with a rapid bolus injection
      b. Weak skeletal muscle relaxant activity
      c. **Antianalgesic** activity (increases sensitivity to pain)
      d. Pharyngeal stimulation
      e. **Very alkaline** solution, which creates problems if improperly administered

  B. Neuroleptanalgesia

    1. **Droperidol and fentanyl** (*Innovar*)
      a. The patient is conscious and can respond.
      b. It can be supplemented with nitrous oxide to induce unconsciousness (neuroleptanesthesia).

    2. **Droperidol** (*Inapsine*), an **antipsychotic drug,** has the following properties:
      a. Antiemetic activity
      b. Extrapyramidal side effects
      c. Reduction of blood pressure due to α-adrenoceptor blockade

    3. **Fentanyl** (*Sublimaze*) and **sufentanil** (*Sufenta*), potent **narcotic analgesics,** have the following properties:
      a. Euphoria
      b. Respiratory depression, which can be reversed by naloxone
      c. Muscle rigidity

    4. The anesthesia is very safe with little cardiovascular depression.

  C. **Ketamine** (*Ketalar*)

    1. This is an analogue of phencyclidine, a hallucinogen.

    2. It induces a **dissociative anesthesia.**

  a. The patient is awake

  b. The analgesic effects are excellent

  c. Muscle tone is either unchanged or increased.

  d. Blood pressure is often increased.

  e. Respiration is not affected.

 3. Ketamine can be administered intravenously or intramuscularly.

 4. **Side effects** are related to hallucinogenic activity, which leads to:

  a. **Vivid dreams**

  b. **Hallucinations,** which can be reduced by diazepam

D. Midazolam (*Versed*)

 1. This is a **water soluble benzodiazepine** with:

  a. A rapid onset of action

  b. A short duration of action

 2. It can induce respiratory depression that is reversible by administration of benzodiazepine antagonists, such as flumazenil (*Mazicon*).

E. Propofol (*Diprivan*)

 1. It has a rapid onset of action.

 2. Although the anesthesia is terminated by redistribution, there are **no cumulative effects** and it can be used for long anesthesias.

 3. The postoperative complications (e.g., nausea, vomiting) are very mild.

IV. LOCAL ANESTHETICS

A. **A reduction of the changes of the** P_{Na} **and** P_K in the activated nerve membrane leads to local anesthesia.

 1. There are no effects on the resting membrane.

 2. The effects on the nerve action potential of both sensory and motor nerve fibers include:

  a. A reduction in the amplitude

  b. A reduction in the rate of rise

  c. A reduction in conduction velocity

  d. A blockade of axonal conduction

 3. Sensory neurons are blocked before motor neurons because the sensory axons are usually smaller and have less myelin.

B. Local anesthetics have 3 common **structural components,** except for benzocaine (Figure 4–1).

 1. The **aromatic** residue is **lipophilic,** which is important for good membrane penetration.

 2. The **amino** group is **hydrophilic.**

  a. It can become charged by picking up a proton.

  b. pH determines whether the local anesthetic is present predominantly in the charged or uncharged forms.

   (1) Only the uncharged form crosses the nerve cell membrane. (Figure 4–2)

   (2) It is converted to the **charged form** inside the axon, which then interacts with binding sites within the ion channels.

   (3) Stock solutions of local anesthetics are acidic (local anesthetic is ionized). The acidity must be neutralized before anesthesia can occur.

Lidocaine

Aromatic residue   Intermediate   Amino group
(lipophilic)   chain   (hydrophilic)

Figure 4-1. General structure of local anesthetics, as illustrated by the amide, lidocaine

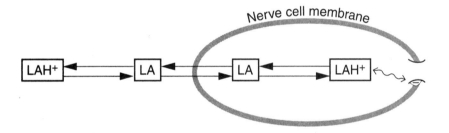

Figure 4-2. The unionized local anesthetic (LA) diffuses across the axon membrane and is converted to the ionized local anesthetic (LAH+), which interacts with binding sites (−) in the sodium and potassium channels.

     (4) Local anesthetics will be less effective for inducing anesthesia in areas of inflammation because:
     (a) The pH is low
     (b) Most of the anesthetic will be charged and unable to penetrate the nerve cell membrane
    (5) Mucous membranes have a low buffering capacity and cannot readily neutralize the acidity of the local anesthetic solution. As a result, mucous membranes are relatively difficult to anesthetize.
  c. The pK_a must be between 7 and 9 so that some of the local anesthetic is present in the charged form and some is present in the uncharged form.

 3. The **intermediate chain** determines how a local anesthetic is metabolized and can be either an ester or an amide.
  a. The **esters** are broken down by butyrylcholinesterases in the blood
    (1) Cocaine is only used for topical anesthesia.
    (2) Procaine (*Novocain*) is metabolized to para-aminobenzoic acid (PABA).
    (3) Chloroprocaine (*Nesacaine*) is metabolized most rapidly, has the shortest duration of action, and theoretically has the lowest risk of systemic toxicity.

(4) Tetracaine (*Pontocaine*) is ten times as potent as procaine and ten times as toxic.

b. The **amides,** which are metabolized by amidases in the liver, include:
(1) Lidocaine (*Xylocaine*)
(2) Mepivacaine (*Carbocaine*)
(3) Bupivacaine (*Marcaine*)

C. **Toxic effects** are very uncommon but can be serious if the systemic absorption of the local anesthetic is excessive.

1. **Myocardial depression** is due to sodium channel blockade in myocardial muscle.

2. **Vasodilation** leads to a fall in blood pressure.

3. **Anxiety or depression and convulsions** result from depressant actions on the CNS.

4. **Hypersensitivity** reactions are rare and occur primarily with esters.

D. **Epinephrine (EPI) is frequently combined with local anesthetics.** It is not used with cocaine, because cocaine by itself has vasoconstrictor activity, and it is not used on end-appendages where ischemia can be induced. EPI reduces blood flow in the anesthetized area which has several effects.

1. **It reduces bleeding,** which is useful during some types of surgeries.

2. **It prolongs the anesthesia** by slowing the loss of anesthetic from the area of injection.

3. **It reduces the systemic concentration** of the anesthetic, thereby lowering the incidence of toxicity.

E. The symptoms of **local anesthetic toxicity must be treated** aggressively.

1. **Oxygen** reduces the hypoxia.

2. **Vasopressors or intravenous fluids** increase the blood pressure.

3. **Diazepam** reduces the convulsions.

F. During spinal anesthesia, blood pressure may fall due to blockade of sympathetic pathways in the spinal cord.

V. SEDATIVE-HYPNOTIC AND ANTIANXIETY DRUGS

A. Hypnotics are medications that induce sleep and antianxiety drugs are medications that reduce anxiety and should have little hypnotic activity.

B. **The common mechanism of action is to enhance the inhibitory effects of gamma-aminobutyric acid (GABA) in the CNS.**

C. **Side effects** common to these drugs include:

1. **Decreased REM sleep** with a rebound increase in REM sleep upon withdrawal

2. **Drowsiness**

3. **Hangover**

4. **Tolerance** with prolonged administration due to:
a. **Increased metabolism** from activation of mixed function oxidases (MFOs)
b. **Reduced effects on the CNS**

5. **Respiratory depression.** These drugs reduce the sensitivity of the medullary respiratory centers to CO_2.

    a. The depression is increased when these drugs are combined with any other sedating drug.

    b. This is the **cause of death** from an overdose.

    c. **Tolerance does not develop to the depressant action on respiration.**

    d. The respiratory depression is very marked with the barbiturates and very weak with the benzodiazepines.

6. **Abuse potential. Physical dependence** occurs with all these drugs and results in an abstinence syndrome upon withdrawal.

D. Benzodiazepines

1. **Antianxiety preparations** usually have long durations of action ranging from twelve hours to several days. They include:

    a. **Chlordiazepoxide** (*Librium*)

    b. **Diazepam** (*Valium*)

    c. **Alprazolam** (*Xanax*)

2. **Hypnotic preparations** (sleeping pills) have shorter durations of action than the antianxiety drugs.

    a. **Flurazepam** (*Dalmane*) has a short half-life, but active metabolites can lead to a long clinical effect, resulting in daytime drowsiness.

    b. **Temazepam** (*Restoril*) has a $t_{1/2}$ of 10 hours with no active metabolites.

    c. **Triazolam** (*Halcion*) has a short $t_{1/2}$ of 2.5 hours, which can result in early morning awakening.

3. **All the benzodiazepines bind to benzodiazepine receptors,** which leads to an enhancement of GABA inhibition (Figure 4–3).

4. **The effects** include:

    a. **Calming** of behavior

    b. **Reduction of anxiety**

    c. **Induction of sleep**

    d. **Anticonvulsant** actions

    e. **Muscle relaxation**

5. There are no autonomic effects.

6. Side effects include:

    a. **Drowsiness**

    b. **Dependence**—long term use should be avoided

    c. **Enhanced depression when combined with other CNS depressant drugs**

7. The benzodiazepines have many **advantages over the barbiturates.**

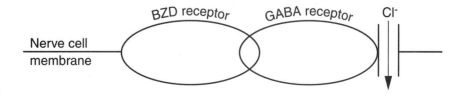

Figure 4-3.   Relationship of the benzodiazepine (BZD) receptor to the gamma-aminobutyric acid (GABA) receptor. Enhanced chloride inflow will hyperpolarize (inhibit) CNS neurons, leading to sedative, antianxiety, and hypnotic effects.

     a. **Abuse is less common,** although it can occur.

     b. **Suicide potential is lower** due to the high therapeutic index (TI).

     c. **Less reduction of REM sleep** occurs.

     d. **The withdrawal syndrome is milder,** although much more prolonged.

     e. **Induction of MFOs is less pronounced.**

     f. **Flumazenil** (*Mazicon*), **a benzodiazepine antagonist,** will reverse the effects of the benzodiazepines.

E. Barbiturates

    1. **Barbituric acid,** a combination of urea and malonic acid, is the basic structural nucleus for these drugs. They are frequently provided as sodium salts (e.g., sodium pentobarbital) because the salt is more water soluble; however, it is very alkaline.

    2. **Durations of action**

     a. **Ultrashort-acting barbiturates** [e.g., thiopental (*Pentothal*)] have very high lipid solubilities due to a sulphur in the structure. They are used as IV anesthetics.

     b. **Short- and intermediate-acting barbiturates** [e.g. pentobarbital (*Nembutal*)] have lower lipid solubilities and longer durations of action that are appropriate for sleeping pills.

     c. **Long-acting barbiturates** [e.g., phenobarbital (*Luminal*)] have the lowest lipid solubilities and the longest durations of action that are appropriate for sedatives or antianxiety drugs.

    3. **Binding to plasma proteins** is highest for the highly lipid-soluble barbiturates.

    4. **Metabolism by side chain oxidation** accounts for the clearance of all the barbiturates from the body. Only phenobarbital has some clearance (30%) by the kidney, and this can be increased by increasing the urinary pH.

    5. **Acute intermittent porphyria is an absolute contraindication** for the use of the barbiturates.

    6. **Symptomatic treatment** is used to manage patients who have overdosed on barbiturates. This includes assisting respiration and stabilizing blood pressure.

F. Chloral hydrate (*Noctec*) **is a hypnotic prodrug** that is metabolized by alcohol dehydrogenase to the active moiety, trichloroethanol.

    1. **An unpleasant taste and odor** reduces the potential for abuse.

    2. **The TI is relatively low.**

G. Buspirone (*BuSpar*) is an antianxiety drug that:

    1. Is not a benzodiazepine

    2. Is a partial agonist at $5HT_{1A}$ receptors.

    3. Does not have any abuse potential

    4. Has few CNS side effects (e.g., drowsiness is minimal)

H. Hydroxyzine (*Atarax, Vistaril*) is an antihistamine with:

    1. Antianxiety activity

    2. No abuse potential

    3. Marked sedative and anticholinergic effects

I. Zolpidem (*Ambien*) is a hypnotic with little effect on the stages of sleep.

J. Clinical uses of sedative–hypnotics and antianxiety drugs include:

1. Treatment of anxiety or neuroses

2. Treatment of insomnia

3. Muscle relaxation

4. Treatment of seizures

5 **Replacement therapy** during withdrawal from sedative–hypnotics (e.g., ethanol)

6. IV anesthesia

7. Sedation before surgical procedures

VI. CNS STIMULANTS

A. Methylxanthines [e.g., caffeine, theophylline (aminophylline), theobromine]

1. The primary **mechanism of action** is controversial.
  a. Adenosine receptors are blocked.
  b. Phosphodiesterases are inhibited at high concentrations which increases the concentration of intracellular cyclic AMP.

2. **Many effects** are induced, including:
  a. CNS stimulation
  b. Myocardial stimulation
  c. Bronchodilation
  d. Diuresis
  e. Constriction of cerebral vessels, which reduces headache

3. Caffeine is more effective on the CNS, and theophylline and theobromine are more effective at the peripheral sites.

B. Amphetamines

1. Absence of a catechol in the structure allows for good penetration into the CNS.

2. The *d*-isomer of amphetamine is more potent on the CNS than the *l*-isomer.

3. Many **effects** occur on the CNS, including:
  a. Improvement of mood
  b. Increase in motor activity
  c. Reduction of appetite which is temporary due to the rapid development of tolerance
  d. Reduction of fatigue

4. **The action is mediated, indirectly,** through the release of endogenous catecholamines.

5. Appropriate indications include
  a. Hyperkinesis in children, especially methylphenidate (*Ritalin*)
  b. Narcolepsy

6. An inappropriate indication is obesity.
  a. Phenylpropanolamine, an amphetamine-like drug, is present in many over-the-counter diet products.
  b. The reduction of appetite is temporary.
  c. Side effects, such as irritability and insomnia, can occur.

C. Convulsants

1. **Picrotoxin is a GABA receptor antagonist** that blocks presynaptic inhibition (Site A in Figure 4–4).

Dorsal neurons

A = Presynaptic inhibitory synapse
B = Postsynaptic inhibitory synapse
C = Excitatory synapse
D = Excitatory synapse
E = Skeletal neuromuscular junction

Skeletal muscle

Ventral motor neuron

Figure 4-4. Neuronal pathways in the spinal cord.

2. Strychnine is a glycine receptor antagonist that blocks postsynaptic inhibition (See Site B in Figure 4–4).

3. Tetanus toxin blocks inhibitory, especially glycine, interneurons.

4. Other convulsants increase excitatory transmission.

5. Their only clinically important effect is respiratory stimulation, but they are not indicated for the treatment of respiratory depression from overdoses of sedative-hypnotics.

VII. ANTIPSYCHOTIC DRUGS

A. The typical antipsychotics **block D_2 dopamine receptors** which accounts for the therapeutic effects of these drugs in reducing the symptoms of many types of psychoses (e.g., schizophrenia).

B. Many other receptors are also blocked which leads to the side effects.

1. Blockade of D_2 receptors in the extrapyramidal system (basal ganglia) induces an iatrogenic parkinsonism.

a. This complication can be reduced by anticholinergic drugs, such as benztropine (*Cogentin*).

b. L-Dopa should not be used to treat antipsychotic-induced extrapyramidal symptoms.

2. Blockade of D_2 receptors in the pituitary enhances the release of prolactin, which induces a **galactorrhea.**

3. Blockade of histamine receptors leads to a **sedation,** but these drugs have no abuse potential and display no tolerance.

4. Blockade of M-cholinoceptors leads to anticholinergic symptoms.

5. Blockade of α-adrenoceptors induces hypotension.

6. Serotonin (5-HT) receptors are also blocked.

7. **An action on the hypothalamus shifts body temperature** towards the ambient temperature.

C. Classes of drugs

    1. Typical drugs
      a. Phenothiazines
        (1) **Chlorpromazine** (*Thorazine*) **and thioridazine** (*Mellaril*) are low potency phenothiazines.
        (2) **Fluphenazine** (*Prolixin*) is a high potency phenothiazine.
      b. Other typical antipsychotics [e.g., **thiothixene** (*Navane*) and **haloperidol** (*Haldol*)] are high potency drugs.

    2. Atypical drugs
      a. **Risperidone** (*Risperdal*) is a new antipsychotic with $5HT_2$ receptor blocking activity and fewer extrapyramidal symptoms than the typical antipsychotics.
      b. **Clozapine** (*Clozaril*) also blocks $5HT_2$ receptors. It:
        (1) Induces the fewest extrapyramidal symptoms
        (2) Is effective in some patients that are refractory to the typical antipsychotic drugs.
        (3) Can cause **agranulocytosis.**
      c. **Olanzapine** (*Zyprexa*) is similar to clozapine, but does not cause agranulocytosis.

    3. Reserpine is an antipsychotic of historical interest only.

D. Side effects

    1. The high potency typical antipsychotics induce the most extrapyramidal symptoms.

    2. The low potency typical antipsychotics induce fewer extrapyramidal symptoms, but they induce more anticholinergic effects, more hypotension, and more sedation than the high potency typical antipsychotics.

    3. **The TI is very large.** At high doses, convulsions can rarely occur.

    4. **Tardive dyskinesia** is a major complication that can develop after long term administration.
      a. **Orofacial** symptoms predominate.
      b. Withdrawal of the antipsychotic drug must be undertaken even though it can enhance the tardive dyskinesia.
      c. Anticholinergics do not reduce the tardive dyskinesia.
      d. One proposed theory is that tardive dyskinesia is due to an **up-regulation of the D_2 receptors** in the basal ganglia.

E. Kinetics

    1. Binding to many tissues results in a **large V_d.**

    2. There are **many drug metabolites.**

    3. The duration of action is very long.

F. Other indications for antipsychotic drugs

    1. They can be used as **antiemetics** because of an action to depress the chemoreceptor trigger zone.

    2. These drugs are used for many less common neurological disorders.

3. These drugs have been used as sedatives, although this is inappropriate in view of the risk of tardive dyskinesia.

VIII. LITHIUM CARBONATE

A. The only clinical indication for lithium is the treatment of **manic depressive illness (bipolar disorder),** including

1. Acute treatment of the manic phase

2. Acute treatment of the depressive phase

3. Prophylaxis

B. A **delay of 7–10 days** occurs before lithium has a clinical effect.

C. **Side effects** are common if the blood lithium concentration gets into the toxic range, thus it is important to monitor the blood lithium concentrations to avoid toxicity.

1. **Tremor** can develop and progress to convulsions.

2. A **nephrogenic diabetes insipidus** can occur.

3. There is **no specific antidote** for lithium.
   a. The thiazide diuretics will lead to lithium retention and enhance lithium toxicity; thus they should be avoided in patients being treated with lithium.
   b. A high sodium diet will increase lithium excretion.

IX. ANTIDEPRESSANTS

A. **Tricyclic antidepressants**

1. Imipramine, the prototype, has a very similar structure to the phenothiazines and many of the effects are similar to the phenothiazines.
   a. The tricyclics produce very **little D_2-receptor antagonism.**
   b. The tricyclics do **reduce amine reuptake,** which increases the concentration of NE and 5-HT in the CNS synapses. This effect does not occur with the phenothiazines.

2. The onset of the antidepressant effect is very slow, taking **2–3 weeks** to develop. This supports a hypothesis that down-regulation of NE or 5-HT receptors may be necessary for the clinical effect to occur.

3. These drugs **improve mood in depressed patients, but not in normal subjects,** which is the basis of the term "antidepressant".

4. **The side effects** vary among specific drugs (Table 4–1), but are generally similar to the phenothiazines. They include:
   a. **Sedation**
   b. **Anticholinergic effects,** such as tachycardia, arrhythmias, and blurred vision
   c. **Antiadrenergic effects,** such as orthostatic hypotension

5. Overdoses from tricyclics are common because depressed patients may ingest large amounts of the drug in an attempt to commit suicide. Treatment of an overdose involves:
   a. Supportive management
   b. Lidocaine to reduce arrhythmias
   c. Physostigmine to reverse anticholinergic effects

6. There are **other clinical uses** for the tricyclics.
   a. **Childhood enuresis** (bed-wetting) and **urinary incontinence** in the elderly can be reduced.
   b. Clomipramine (*Anafranil*) reduces obsessive-compulsive behaviors.

Table 4-1

Magnitude of Side Effects from Tricyclic Antidepressants

	Sedation and anticholinergic activity
Doxepin (*Sinequan*)	High
Amitriptyline (*Elavil*)	High
Imipramine (*Tofranil*)	Moderate
Desipramine (*Norpramin*)	Low
Nortriptyline (*Aventyl, Pamelor*)	Low

B. Selective serotonin reuptake inhibitors (SSRIs)

1. Most new antidepressants, such as **fluoxetine** (*Prozac*), **sertraline** (*Zoloft*) and **paroxetine** (*Paxil*), inhibit serotonin reuptake but do not affect NE reuptake.

2. This class of drugs is very effective in the treatment of depression.

3. The main advantage is they are **much safer** due to a lack of:
a. Sedation
b. Hypotension
c. Anticholinergic effects

4. They can cause CNS stimulation, leading to **insomnia.**

C. Monoamine oxidase (MAO) inhibitors

1. Tranylcypromine (*Parnate*) and phenelzine (*Nardil*) are **competitive irreversible inhibitors of both MAO$_A$ and MAO$_B$.** This inhibition increases the concentrations of NE and other amines in the granules, which increases amine release.

2. The MAO inhibitors **elevate mood in both normal and depressed people.**

3. **The side effects** can be severe, including:
a. Hepatotoxicity
b. CNS stimulation
c. Postural hypotension
d. Hypertensive crisis from
(1) Foods containing tyramine, such as cheeses, beans, pickled herring, beer, and wine
(2) Over-the-counter sympathomimetics

4. Combinations of tricyclics and MAO inhibitors should be avoided because this can lead to excessive CNS stimulation.

X. DRUGS FOR PARKINSON'S DISEASE

A. **Parkinson's disease is due to a reduced dopamine (DA) content** in the cells of the **substantia nigra,** which leads to the symptoms of:

1. Tremor at rest

2. Cogwheel rigidity

3. Akinesia

4. Loss of postural reflexes

B. **Methylphenyltetrahydropyridine (MPTP) destroys DA neurons** and induces parkinsonian symptoms. This can be used to produce a valuable animal model.

C. Many **treatments** are available for Parkinson's disease, which either increase DA effects or block ACh in the basal ganglia.

1. Levodopa [L-dopa(*Dopar,Larodopa*)] is metabolized by dopa decarboxylase to DA, which increases the availability of DA, an inhibitory transmitter, in the basal ganglia.

    a. The L-dopa is effective in a few weeks, especially **for reducing the rigidity and akinesia.**

    b. There are **problems** with L-dopa therapy.

        (1) L-Dopa is **rapidly metabolized** in peripheral tissues, so that only 1% of the administered dose reaches the CNS.

        (2) Pyridoxine (vitamin B_6) increases this metabolism by activating dopa decarboxylase.

    c. L-Dopa is usually combined with carbidopa (*Sinemet*), **a peripheral dopa decarboxylase inhibitor.** The L-dopa dosage can then be reduced by 80% without changing the effectiveness. The side effects from conversion of L-dopa to DA in the periphery are also reduced.

    d. The side effects from L-dopa are quite prominent.

        (1) Nausea, vomiting, and anorexia induced by stimulation of the chemoreceptor trigger zone can limit the usefulness of this treatment. The severity of the nausea is reduced by gradually increasing the dose into the therapeutic range and by combining L-dopa with carbidopa.

        (2) Postural hypotension can occur.

        (3) Arrhythmias can develop from actions of DA on the heart.

        (4) Choreiform movements are indicative of excessive basal ganglion activity.

        (5) Psychological disturbances can lead to insomnia and delirium.

    e. ON-OFF effects often develop after a year or more. These are indicative of "wearing off phenomena" at the end of dosage intervals and erratic effectiveness.

    f. Contraindications for L-dopa include:

        (1) Treatment with MAO inhibitors, because the combination can lead to a hypertensive crisis

        (2) Glaucoma, because L-dopa can induce a mydriasis

        (3) Psychiatric disorders, especially those disorders being treated with antipsychotic drugs, which are DA antagonists.

2. Bromocriptine (*Parlodel*) and **pergolide** (*Permax*) are **DA receptor agonists** that have many effects and side effects that are similar to L-dopa. They are often used with L-dopa and carbidopa to reduce the ON-OFF effects.

3. The anticholinergics [e.g., trihexyphenidyl (*Artane*), benztropine (*Cogentin*)] reduce the cholinergic excitatory tone in the basal ganglia.

    a. They are most frequently used in combination **with antipsychotic drugs** to reduce the extrapyramidal symptoms from the antipsychotic drugs.

    b. The side effects are due to central and peripheral cholinoceptor blockade.

4. Amantadine (*Symmetrel*) is an anti-viral drug that reduces the symptoms of Parkinson's disease. Tolerance to this therapeutic effect often develops within 6 months.

5. Antihistamines, such as diphenhydramine (*Benadryl*), do have some weak therapeutic effects which are probably due to the anticholinergic actions of these drugs.

6. Selegiline (*Eldepryl*) is a MAO_B inhibitor.

    a. A slowing of the metabolism of DA enhances the effectiveness of L-dopa.

    b. It may also slow the onset of Parkinson's disease when given alone by reducing the activation of a toxic environmental substance (by MAO_B) that is responsible for the disease.

D. The order of efficacies of the available drugs for this disease is the following: L-dopa > bromocriptine > amantadine > anticholinergics

E. A common approach is to use the low efficacy drugs (e.g., selegiline, amantadine, anticholinergics) during the early stages of Parkinson's disease and reserve L-dopa with carbidopa and dopaminergic agonists for the later stages.

XI. DRUGS FOR HUNTINGTON'S DISEASE

A. **A loss of GABA or increased DA** in the basal ganglia leads to the choreiform movements. As a result, L-dopa and anticholinergics are inappropriate treatments.

B. **No treatment is very effective,** but some reduction of symptoms can be induced by DA depleters, antipsychotics (DA blockers) or cholinesterase inhibitors.

XII. ANTICONVULSANTS

A. **Animal models** are useful in the screening of potential drugs for the treatment of epilepsy.

   1. **The convulsant, pentylenetetrazol,** induces convulsions that have drug sensitivities similar to absence seizures.

   2. **Maximal electrical shock** induces convulsions with drug sensitivities similar to tonic-clonic seizures.

   3. **Kindling** from weak, long-term stimulation of the cortex or amygdala induces generalized seizures.

B. These **drugs act by reducing the excitability** of focal and **non-focal neurons** (primarily).

   1. **Enhancement of GABA inhibition** leads to an increased P_{Cl} and a hyperpolarization of neuronal membranes.

   2. All sedative-hypnotic and antianxiety drugs have anticonvulsant activity, but most produce too much drowsiness (sedation) to be clinically useful.

C. **The selection** of a specific drug for treatment depends upon the **seizure type** (Table 4–2).

D. Each anticonvulsant has some unique features.

   1. **Phenobarbital** (*Luminal*) has a half-life of 4 days. Patients develop some tolerance to the sedative-hypnotic effect, but not to the anti-epileptic effect.

   2. **Primidone** (*Mysoline*) is an active drug and is also partially metabolized to phenobarbital, thus it has properties that are very similar to phenobarbital.

Table 4-2
Activities of Anticonvulsants for Specific Seizure Patterns

	Tonic-clonic	Partial	Absence	Akinetic and atonic
Phenobarbital (*Luminal*)	+	+		
Primidone (*Mysoline*)	+	+		
Phenytoin (*Dilantin*)	++	++	⊖	
Carbamazepine (*Tegretol*)	++	++		
Valproic acid (*Depakene*)	+	+	++	+
Ethosuximide (*Zarontin*)			++	
Clonazepam (*Klonopin*)			+	+

Note: (–) means exacerbated

3. Phenytoin (*Dilantin*) is an effective anti-epileptic with no sedative activity.
   a. **Elimination follows zero-order kinetics.**
   b. **Gingival hyperplasia and cardiac arrhythmias** are important side effects.

4. Carbamazepine (*Tegretol*) is a tricyclic anticonvulsant which has **antidepressant** activity. A rare, but severe, side effect is **aplastic anemia.**

5. Valproic acid (*Depakene*) is useful for **many types of seizures.** It can be **hepato-toxic.**

6. Ethosuximide (*Zarontin*) is the drug of choice for **absence seizures.**

7. Clonazepam (*Klonopin*) is a benzodiazepine, which produces considerable sedation.

8. Gabapentin (*Neurontin*) is useful for partial seizures.

E. Many features are common to most antiepileptics.

   1. None of these drugs are curative.

   2. They tend to be **highly bound to plasma proteins.**

   3. They are usually **cleared by hepatic metabolism.**
      a. They may **inhibit the metabolism** of other drugs.
      b. They may **induce the metabolism** of other drugs.
      c. It is important to measure the serum anticonvulsant concentration.

   4. Side effects that usually occur, include:
      a. **CNS depression** (Even phenytoin induces a lethargy.)
      b. **Skin rashes**
      c. **Nystagmus**
      d. **Teratogenicity**

F. **Treatment of status epilepticus** must be initiated rapidly.

   1. **An intravenous benzodiazepine,** such as diazepam, is the treatment of choice.

   2. If the benzodiazepine is ineffective, other measures must be tried, including:
      a. **Phenytoin, given intravenously**
      b. **Phenobarbital, given intravenously**
      c. **General anesthesia**

XIII. ANALGESIC ANTIPYRETICS

A. All the analgesic antipyretics act by **inhibiting cyclooxygenase (COX)** which reduces prostaglandin synthesis.

B. Aspirin and other salicylates

   1. Aspirin (acetylsalicylic acid) acetylates and irreversibly inhibits COX-1 and COX-2. New COX must be synthesized to recover from the effects of aspirin.

   2. The major **therapeutic effects** include:
      a. **Mild analgesia,** due to reduced prostaglandin synthesis at the sensory nerve endings.
      b. **Antipyresis,** due to reduced prostaglandin synthesis in the hypothalamic temperature control center. This reduces an elevated body temperature.
      c. **Anti-inflammatory** actions at high doses, due to reduced prostaglandins at the sites of inflammation.

   3. These effects occur without tolerance and without euphoria.

   4. There are many **side effects** from aspirin, including:

   a. Gastric ulcerations and gastric hemorrhaging

   b. **Inhibition of platelet aggregation.** This adverse effect is taken advantage of during the management of patients:

     (1) After a myocardial infarction

     (2) With transient ischemic attacks

     (3) With angina, especially unstable angina

   c. **Hypersensitivity** reactions that:

     (1) Are not immunologically mediated

     (2) May be due to increased **leukotrienes**

   d. **Reduced renal uric acid secretion at low doses** and reduced uric acid reabsorption (uricosuria) at high doses

   e. **Reye's syndrome** in children with chicken pox (varicella) or influenza viral infections. Aspirin is best avoided in children.

5. Aspirin induces many **toxic effects** which occur in the following order as the dose is increased from the therapeutic range to the toxic range.

   a. **Tinnitus** is an early indicator of toxicity.

   b. **Uncoupling of oxidative phosphorylation** increases CO_2 production, which increases respiration.

   c. **Direct medullary stimulation** also enhances respiration, leading to respiratory alkalosis and HCO_3 excretion (loss).

   d. **Acidosis** subsequently occurs as a result of:

     (1) **Direct respiratory depression**

     (2) **Acidic products** of aspirin metabolism. This leads to a fluid and electrolyte loss.

     (3) **Previous loss of HCO_3**

6. **Management** of aspirin overdoses involves:

   a. **Emesis or lavage**

   b. **Fluids with HCO_3**

   c. **Monitoring the blood aspirin concentration** beginning 6 hours after ingestion

C. Acetaminophen (*Tylenol*)

1. The primary **effects** of acetaminophen are quite different from aspirin, and include:

   a. **Mild analgesic activity**

   b. **Antipyretic activity**

   c. **No anti-inflammatory activity**

   d. **None of the side effects of aspirin**

2. **The major adverse effect** from high doses is a **delayed hepatic necrosis.**

   a. A toxic phase 1 metabolite builds up in the liver because of the **depletion of glutathione.**

   b. This toxicity is especially prominent in combination with ethanol.

   c. The hepatotoxicity can be avoided by early administration of **N-acetylcysteine,** which replenishes the stores of glutathione.

D. Ibuprofen (*Motrin*, *Nuprin*, *Advil*) and **naproxen** (*Aleve*)

1. The effects of ibuprofen and naproxen are very **similar to aspirin,** including

   a. **Mild analgesic activity.** Ibuprofen is especially effective for dysmenorrhea.

   b. **Antipyretic activity**

   c. **Anti-inflammatory activity**

2. **The side effects** are similar to, but milder than, the side effects for aspirin, including:

    a Gastrointestinal bleeding

    b. Increased bleeding times

    c. Overdose toxicity like aspirin

E. Ketorolac (*Toradol*)

    1. This is an unusual NSAID, in that it can be **given intramuscularly** as well as orally.

    2. It is only used for the **treatment of acute pain,** and has a clinical efficacy similar to morphine.

XIV. NARCOTIC ANALGESICS

A. **The prototype, morphine,** is extracted from the opium poppy in which 10% of the alkaloid content is morphine and 1% is codeine.

B. Morphine and codeine can be modified to form semisynthetic derivatives, including:

    1. Heroin (diacetylmorphine), which is more lipid soluble and has a more rapid onset of action

    2. Oxycodone (*Roxicodone*)

    3. Levorphanol (*Levo-Dromoran*)

C. Many synthetic narcotics have also been produced, such as:

    1. Meperidine (*Demerol*)

    2. Methadone (*Dolophine*)

    3. Fentanyl (*Sublimaze*)

    4. Propoxyphene (*Darvon,Dolene*)

D. **The properties** of morphine are representative of most of the drugs in this class.

    1. **The kinetics** of morphine are well explored.

        a. **Absorption from the gut** is good, but the serum morphine concentration is **variable** due to first-pass metabolism by the liver.

        b. It is **metabolized by glucuronide conjugation.**

        c. Parenteral administration is commonly used to induce a rapid, predictable analgesic effect.

        d. The drug distributes in the total body water.

    2. **The binding sites** for morphine are the endorphin, dynorphin, and enkephalin receptors. **Mu, kappa and delta receptor subtypes** have been identified.

    3. Morphine induces many pharmacological **effects.**

        a. **Analgesia** occurs due to a decrease of pain perception and a decrease in the psychological response to pain.

            (1) An **inhibitory** action **on substance P release** in the spinal cord has been described (Figure 4–5), which may account for some of the analgesic effects.

            (2) This is accompanied by a **mental clouding** or drowsiness.

            (3) Although the first dose can be dysphoric, subsequent doses produce a euphoria.

        b. **Respiratory depression** is induced by a reduction in the sensitivity of the medullary respiratory centers to CO_2. This occurs with all the narcotic analgesics and is the primary **cause of death** from an acute overdose.

  c. **Physical dependence and tolerance** occur, which means that a withdrawal syndrome will develop when the drug is discontinued. Cross-tolerance occurs with all other narcotic analgesics.

  d. **Antitussive** (cough suppressant) actions are prominent.

  e. **An emetic action** is often observed with the initial doses.

  f. **Miosis** is induced by increased parasympathetic tone to the pupil. This is less pronounced with meperidine due to an anticholinergic effect.

  g. **Constipation** results from decreased GI motility, even though there is an increased tone of the GI smooth muscle.

  h. **Histamine release** can be induced.

  i. **Increased tone of the biliary tract and ureters** also occurs.

E. **Narcotic antagonists** have a structure that is very similar to morphine (Figure 4–6). A bulky substitution on the nitrogen results in antagonistic activity.

  1. **The pure antagonists** have no analgesic activity.

    a. **Naloxone** (*Narcan*) and **naltrexone** (*Trexan*) will:

      (1) **Reverse the respiratory depression** from an overdose of a narcotic

      (2) Not affect the respiratory depression from a sedative-hypnotic

      (3) **Induce a withdrawal syndrome** in a narcotic addict

    b. **Naltrexone is more effective orally** and has a **longer duration of action** than naloxone.

  2. **The weak agonist/antagonist (partial agonist) analgesics,** such as **pentazocine** (*Talwin*), have analgesic activity in addition to antagonistic activity; thus they are partial agonists.

    a. They **will not reverse the respiratory depression** caused by a narcotic.

    b. They will **induce a withdrawal syndrome** in a narcotic addict.

    c. Most new narcotic analgesics are in this group. The rationale behind their use

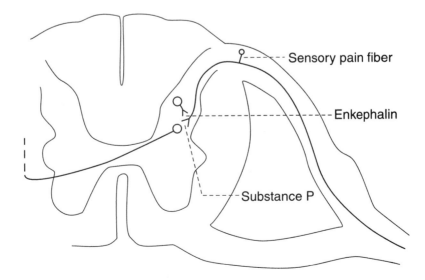

Figure 4-5.   Presynaptic inhibition by enkephalins on substance P release in the spinal pain pathway.

is that these analgesics should be abused less and should have less respiratory depression.

F. **Therapeutic uses** of the narcotic analgesics include:

1. Analgesia
   a. Morphine is more potent than codeine, which is more potent than aspirin.
   b. Narcotics are used primarily for short term analgesia (e.g., myocardial infarction), except in terminal patients. The analgesic antipyretics are preferred to reduce chronic pain.

2. **Diarrhea. Diphenoxylate** with atropine (*Lomotil*) or **loperamide** (*Imodium*) are preferred as they have few CNS effects.

3. **Neuroleptic anesthesia** (e.g., fentanyl)

4. **Antitussive** activity
   a. **Codeine** induces more cough suppression than morphine.
   b. **Dextromethorphan** (*Benylin DM*) has little narcotic activity, but it does have cough suppressant activity.

5. **Reduction of narcotic withdrawal symptoms.** This requires a drug, such as **methadone,** with a long duration of action.

6. **Maintenance of a narcotic addict,** using methadone

G. **Clinical uses of the narcotic antagonists** include:

1. **Analgesia** with the agonist/antagonist analgesics

2. **Treatment of the respiratory depression from an acute narcotic overdose** using naloxone

3. **Diagnosis of physical dependence** to a narcotic. Naloxone will precipitate an abstinence syndrome in narcotic addicts.

4. **Management of a narcotic addict.** Naltrexone will reduce the euphoric effects of the narcotics.

Figure 4-6. Modification of the narcotic structure (at N) results in the narcotic antagonists. This diagram shows the structure of morphine.

5

Substance Abuse

I. GENERAL FEATURES

A. Abuse of a drug is often, but not always, associated with kinetic, dynamic, homeostatic or learned **tolerance.**

B. An acute tolerance (with first dose) has been described for ethanol.

C. **Cross-tolerance** occurs between drugs with the same mechanism of action.

D. Repeated drug use may also lead to **psychological dependence, physical dependence and cross-dependence** (between drugs with the same mechanism of action).

E. The symptoms during withdrawal tend to mirror (be the opposite of) those from drug administration.

F. Withdrawal from a drug of abuse is usually less severe with long-acting drugs than with short-acting drugs. This is the theoretical basis for replacement therapy.

G. Abusers of drugs usually derive more pleasure from a drug with a rapid onset of action than from a drug with a slow onset of action within the same class.

II. SEDATIVE-HYPNOTICS

A. Ethanol

1. Due to **high lipid solubility and high water solubility,** ethanol distributes in the total body water.

2. **Clearance** from the body involves metabolism by the liver.

    a. **Metabolism** by the **alcohol and aldehyde dehydrogenases** (Figure 5–1) follows zero-order kinetics.

        (1) The products are acetaldehyde and acetic acid.

        (2) Two molecules of NADH are produced for each molecule of ethanol.

    b. An insignificant amount is metabolized by mixed function oxidases (MFOs), but this induces the MFOs.

3. The effects of ethanol are related to the blood ethanol concentration.

    a. **The legal limit** for driving in most states is **100 mg% (100 mg/100 ml).**

    b. **Death** can occur in the range of **500 mg%,** although this is quite variable.

    c. **Treatment** of an overdose of ethanol is **symptomatic.**

4. **Acute adverse effects** can be produced by a single exposure to ethanol.

    a. **Behavior is changed** due to a loss of inhibitions.

    b. The effects of other CNS depressants are enhanced.

    c. **Hypothermia** results from a peripheral vasodilation, which makes a person feel warm even though body heat is being lost.

    d. **Hangovers** are common after drinking ethanol, and may represent symptoms of an acute withdrawal.

Figure 5-1. Metabolism of ethanol. *NAD*=nicotinamide adenine dinucleotide; *NADH*=reduced nicotinamide adenine dinucleotide

> **5.** **Adverse effects from chronic (repeated) use** occur on almost every tissue in the body and include:
>   **a.** **Physical and psychological dependence**
>   **b.** **Activation of MFOs,** which increases the metabolism of many other drugs (e.g., phenytoin, warfarin)
>   **c.** **Edema**
>   **d.** **Hypertension**
>   **e.** **Cardiomyopathy**
>   **f.** **Liver damage** (e.g., cirrhosis)
>   **g.** **Changes in blood glucose**
>   **h.** **Damage to the gastrointestinal tract**
>   **i.** **Anemias**
>   **j.** **Malnutrition, especially thiamine deficiency** which leads to the Wernicke-Korsakoff syndrome
>   **k.** **Psychological depression**
>   **l.** **Fetal alcohol syndrome,** which is a common cause of birth defects
>
> **6.** A low intake of ethanol (one drink per day) increases HDL and decreases LDL cholesterol. This may reduce the risk of heart disease.
>
> **7.** **Withdrawal** from ethanol in someone who is dependent leads to a **stimulatory syndrome** which lasts about one week.
>   **a.** **Tremor, hallucinations, convulsions and delirium tremens** can occur during withdrawal.
>   **b.** It is important to **replace thiamine** and improve the diet.
>   **c.** The severity of the withdrawal symptoms can be reduced by **replacement therapy with an antianxiety drug** (e.g., diazepam or chlordiazepoxide).
>
> **8.** Long-term treatment of a recovering alcoholic requires counseling and group support therapy.
>
> **9.** **Disulfiram** (*Antabuse*) is occasionally useful to help alcoholics avoid the use of ethanol.
>   **a.** It inhibits the enzyme, **aldehyde dehydrogenase.**
>   **b.** **An accumulation of acetaldehyde** leads to a toxic syndrome whenever ethanol is ingested.
>
> **10.** **Methanol** has intoxicating effects similar to ethanol, except it is much more toxic.
>   **a.** Metabolism by alcohol and aldehyde dehydrogenases results in the production of **formaldehyde and formic acid.**
>   **(1)** **Acidosis** is the cause of death from acute ingestion.
>   **(2)** **Retinal nerve damage** leads to blindness.

      b. **The specific antidote** for the treatment of methanol intoxication is **ethanol,** which competes with methanol at the metabolic enzymes and slows the production of the toxic metabolites.

    11. **Ethylene glycol** is metabolized by the same pathway to products which cause acidosis and renal failure. An acute intoxication is treated in a manner similar to methanol intoxication.

B. Barbiturates

    1. **Pentobarbital and secobarbital** are very common drugs of abuse, although any sedative-hypnotic or antianxiety drug can be abused.

    2. These drugs produce a **CNS depression with euphoria,** reduction of anxiety, and drowsiness, which is similar to the effects of ethanol.
        a. **Tolerance** occurs, but it is not large (5–10 times)
        b. **Cross-tolerance** develops to alcohol, barbiturates, general anesthetics, benzodiazepines, and other sedative-hypnotics.

    3. An overdose leads to **respiratory depression,** which should be treated symptomatically.

    4. **Barbiturate withdrawal can be severe** and life-threatening with:
        a. **A prolonged delirium**
        b. **Grand mal convulsions**

    5. **Substitution therapy** (e.g., phenobarbital, given orally) can be used to reduce the withdrawal symptoms. The phenobarbital is then slowly withdrawn.

C. Benzodiazepines

    1. These drugs have effects that are similar to other sedative-hypnotics, although they are less subject to abuse than the barbiturates.

    2. When they are abused, the withdrawal syndrome is very mild, but very long in duration.

D. Inhalants

    1. Inhalation of vapors from solvents, glue, gasoline, or anesthetics induces effects that are also very similar to ethanol.

    2. Use of inhalants is most common in very young abusers.

    3. As with other halogenated hydrocarbons, hepatotoxicity, cardiac toxicity, and carcinogenicity can occur.

III. OPIOIDS

A. **Heroin, used intravenously,** is the most popular opioid for abuse.

B. The initial dose may be unpleasant with nausea, but subsequent doses induce euphoria in the abuser.

C. **Marked tolerance** (up to 1000 times) to the desired effects occurs with repeated use of the opioids.

D. **Common causes of death** in heroin addicts are:

    1. **Respiratory depression** from an overdose. This can be reversed with naloxone.

    2. **Infections** from using unsterilized needles and syringes

E. The withdrawal syndrome begins in 6 hours and peaks in 48 hours.

F. **Withdrawal** from heroin can be performed by:

1. **"Cold turkey"** (provide only symptomatic treatment)

2. **Replacement therapy with methadone**

3. **Treatment with clonidine** to reduce the symptoms

G. After withdrawal, abusers need long-term **rehabilitation** with

1. **Group therapy**

2. **Methadone maintenance,** which induces tolerance so no effect is obtained from heroin

3. **Depot naltrexone**

IV. CIGARETTES

A. **Nicotine** is the active substance and is responsible for the addictive nature of cigarettes.

1. **Stimulation of CNS** induces arousal, relaxation, and a mild euphoria.

2. **Activation of the sympathetic nervous system** induces a vasoconstriction and an increase in blood pressure.

B. **The tars and carbon monoxide** inhaled increase the risk of:

1. **Chronic obstructive pulmonary disease (COPD)**

2. **Cancer**

3. **Heart disease**

C. **Physical and psychological dependence** occurs. Abstinence leads to anxiety, insomnia, and enhanced appetite which can last for several months.

D. Many approaches are available which slightly increase the probability of successfully abstaining from cigarettes.

1. Nicotine is available in a patch, in gum, and in an inhaler.

2. Bupropion (*Zyban*) is an antidepressant that has been introduced as an aid to stop smoking.

3. Behavioral modification programs are also helpful.

V. CNS STIMULANTS

A. **Cocaine and amphetamines** are the most commonly abused CNS stimulants.

B. The magnitude of the euphoria depends on the speed of onset.

1. **Amphetamines** are usually taken orally, which results in a **slow onset.**

2. Cocaine can be ingested, chewed, snorted, injected, or smoked (as crack in the free base form). **Crack** that is smoked has the most **rapid onset** and induces the most pleasurable effects.

C. They produce a **euphoria** with:

1. **Little physical dependence.** Fatigue is the primary physical symptom during withdrawal.

2. **Strong psychological dependence.**

D. The period of euphoria varies depending on the half-life of the drug in the body.

    1. **Cocaine induces** a **very short euphoria** (approximately 15 minutes) that is followed by a period of **marked dysphoria.**

    2. The euphoria from amphetamines has a much longer duration.

E. Chronic abusers develop **paranoid, psychotic-like** symptoms.

F. **Overdoses** can be dangerous.

    1. **Sympathomimetic actions** can lead to **tachycardia and arrhythmias.**

    2. Abusers can become **aggressive** and experience **hallucinations.**

    3. **Cocaine** can also induce:
        a. **Gangrene,** due to a peripheral vasoconstriction
        b. **Perforation of the nasal septum,** due to vasoconstriction in the nasal mucosa
        c. **Convulsions,** due to local anesthetic effects on the brain

VI. HALLUCINOGENS

A. These are drugs that **induce visual hallucinations.**

    1. **Lysergic acid diethylamide (LSD),** psilocin, and harmaline are examples of **indole** hallucinogens.
        a. The indole structure in these substances also occurs in serotonin.
        b. They may act by blocking serotonin receptors.

    2. **Mescaline** is a **phenylethylamine** hallucinogen. The phenylethylamines have more **sympathomimetic** effects than the indoles.

    3. **No physical dependence** occurs.

    4. **Cross-tolerance** occurs between the indole and phenylethylamine hallucinogens.

    5. Overdoses can result in a state of panic and psychotic behavior. These symptoms can be treated with diazepam.

B. Phencyclidine (PCP)

    1. PCP, or "angel dust," is structurally similar to the anesthetic ketamine.

    2. Although it produces hallucinations, there is **no cross-tolerance with LSD.**

    3. Low doses induce a **drunken-like state.**

    4. High doses produce an **amphetamine-like state** in which the abuser can become very physically aggressive and difficult to control; thus it is a very dangerous drug.

VII. MARIJUANA

A. **The hemp plant** is the source of marijuana, which contains the active ingredient, Δ^9**tetrahydrocannabinol (Δ^9THC).** It is usually abused by smoking.

    1. Δ^9THC is **very lipid soluble** and traces remain in the body for days after use.

    2. **Metabolism** to an active product, 11-OH-Δ^9THC, occurs in the liver. This product is further hydroxylated to an inactive metabolite, 8,11-OH$_2$-Δ^9THC.

B. **A vivid dream-like state** is induced with some **motor incoordination** and a **loss of sense of time.** Hallucinations can occur at high doses.

C. Chronic use leads to **some tolerance** for these effects, **apathy, and chronic bronchitis.**

D. **Dronabinol** (*Marinol*), which is Δ^9THC, has **antiemetic** activity that is useful during cancer chemotherapy.

6

Autacoids, Drugs for Inflammatory Disorders, and Vitamins

I. HISTAMINE

A. Histamine is present in mast cells and circulating basophils, and it is an autacoid. Autacoids are substances that function as local hormones or neuromodulators in the body.

B. Histamine **acts on H_1 and H_2 receptors** at many sites in the body.

    1. The important pharmacological effects of histamine are listed in Table 6–1.

    2. A **triple response** is induced after intradermal injection.

        a. A **direct vasodilation** produces a localized **red spot** at the site of injection.

        b. **Activation of nerve endings** induces an axon reflex that produces a vasodilation and a **flare**.

        c. **Increased capillary permeability** induces a **wheal**.

C. The **clinical uses** of histamine are of minor importance.

    1. **Testing for achlorhydria** after administration of histamine is useful for diagnosing **pernicious anemia**. The treatment for pernicious anemia is **vitamin B_{12} (cyanocobalamin)**.

    2. Supersensitivity to histamine can be useful for the **diagnosis of asthma.**

D. Betazole is a selective H_2 agonist, which acts primarily to increase gastric secretions.

II. HISTAMINE BLOCKERS

A. Many allergic disorders can be treated with histamine blockers.

B. The effects of endogenous histamine release can be blocked by several classes of drugs.

    1. **Cromolyn** (*Intal*) **reduces mast cell degranulation.**

        a. The release of all mast cell mediators, including histamine, is decreased.

        b. **Inhalation** of the dry powder or aerosol is the usual route of administration, because cromolyn is not absorbed after oral administration.

        c. The primary clinical use of cromolyn is the **prophylactic treatment of asthma and allergic disorders.**

    2. H_1 **antihistamines are competitive antagonists** at H_1 receptors. Drugs in this class include diphenhydramine (*Benadryl*), dimenhydrinate (*Dramamine*) and chlorpheniramine (*Chlor-Trimeton, Teldrin*).

        a. On-going histamine effects are only weakly reduced, thus the H_1-antihistamines work best if administered before exposure to an allergen.

Table 6–1
Effects of Histamine

Receptors	Effects
H_1 & H_2	Vasodilates arterioles and venules (leads to hypotension and shock)
H_1 & H_2	Increases capillary permeability (leads to edema)
H_1	Contracts bronchial and intestinal smooth muscle
H_1	Acts on sensory nerve endings to cause pain and itching
H_2	Increases heart rate and contractility
H_2	Increases gastric secretions

    b. The activity versus acute allergic reactions is better than the activity versus chronic allergies.

    c. There are many **clinical uses** for H_1 antihistamines, including treatment of:
        (1) Seasonal allergic rhinitis
        (2) Acute urticaria
        (3) Anxiety
        (4) Insomnia
        (5) Nausea
        (6) Parkinson's disease

    d. The **side effects** include:
        (1) Sedation
        (2) **Anticholinergic symptoms,** such as constipation, urinary retention, and dry mouth

    e. The second-generation H_1-antihistamines [e.g., loratadine (*Claritin*)] do not have these side effects.

  3. The **H_2 antihistamines** [e.g., cimetidine (*Tagamet*)] act primarily to reduce gastric secretions and are used to treat **peptic ulcer disease** (See Chapter 2 XII A 2). They have no effects on H_1 receptors.

III. EICOSANOIDS

  A. This large group of autacoids is **widely distributed** in the body.

  B. They are locally synthesized (Figure 6–1) and released as needed **(de novo synthesis).**

  C. The synthesis of prostacyclin (PGI_2), prostaglandins and thromboxane (TXA_2) is reduced by aspirin and the NSAIDs, which inhibit the enzyme cyclooxygenase. The NSAIDs have no effect on lipoxygenase.

  D. The eicosanoids have very **short durations** of action (approximately 1 minute) and induce **many effects.**

    1. Prostaglandin E_2 (PGE_2) or dinoprostone (*Prostin E2*) and $PGF_{2\alpha}$ or carboprost (*Prostin 15M*) **increase uterine activity.**
      a. They can be used to **induce labor and abortions.**
      b. Ibuprofen, by blocking prostaglandin synthesis, reduces the symptoms of dysmenorrhea.

    2. Prostaglandin E_1 (PGE_1) or alprostadil (*Prostin VR*) can be used to relax vascular smooth muscle and **maintain a patent ductus arteriosus.** Indomethacin, by blocking prostaglandin synthesis, induces closure of the ductus arteriosus.

    3. PGE **bronchodilates** and PGF **bronchoconstricts.**

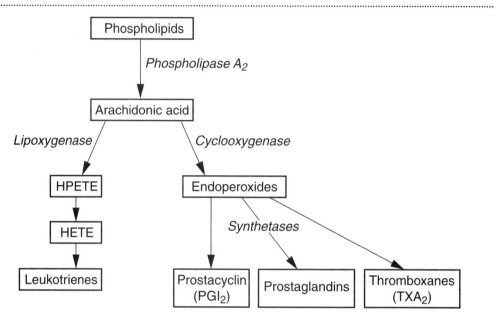

Figure 6–1. Synthesis of the eicosanoids. *HPETE*=hydroperoxyeicosatetraenoic acid; *HETE*=hydroxy-eicosatetraenoic acid

4. PGE and PGI$_2$ **decrease gastric acid secretions. Misoprostol** (*Cytotec*) is a PGE$_1$ derivative that is used to **reduce gastric ulcerations from the NSAIDs.**

5. PGE and PGI$_2$ **sensitize afferent nerve endings to pain.**

6. Eicosanoids have many circulatory effects.
   a. TXA$_2$ from platelets and PGI$_2$ from vessel walls are important local hormones in the **control of the microcirculation** (Figure 6–2).
   b. PGI$_2$ or epoprostenol (*Flolan*) vasodilates and can be administered from an IV infusion pump to **treat primary pulmonary hypertension.**
   c. Alprostadil injected into the penis causes a vasodilation and induces a **penile erection.**

IV. DRUGS FOR MIGRAINE HEADACHES

A. An initial intracranial vasoconstriction is followed by a prolonged extracranial vasodilation during which the migraine headache occurs.

B. Acute treatment

   1. **Mild analgesics** can be used for weak migraines.

   2. **Ergotamine,** often combined with caffeine (*Cafergot*), induces a **direct vasoconstriction.** It is only used acutely because of the toxicity (e.g., prolonged vasoconstriction can result in gangrene) associated with chronic administration.

   3. **Sumatriptan** (*Imitrex*) **vasoconstricts by activating 5-HT$_1$ receptors.** Although safer than ergotamine, there is a risk of inducing a coronary vasospasm in patients with coronary artery disease.

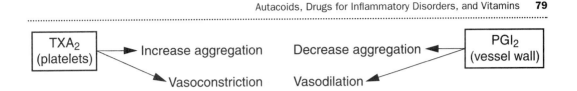

Figure 6–2. Local hormonal control of the microcirculation by thromboxane (TXA_2) in the platelets and prostacyclin (PGI_2) in the vessel wall.

C. Prophylaxis

1. The **β-blockers and calcium channel blockers** are effective.

2. Methysergide (*Sansert*), **a partial 5-HT agonist,** has a delayed onset, but can be used for prophylaxis.

V. ANTIASTHMATIC DRUGS

A. Asthma appears to be caused by an **inflammation of the airways** with **bronchoconstriction, bronchial wall edema, and increased respiratory secretions.**

B. **Methacholine and histamine** induce a bronchoconstriction and can be used as **provocative** diagnostic tests for asthma, although this can be dangerous.

C. **The sympathomimetics** relieve the acute symptoms of asthma by **$β_2$-mediated bronchodilation** and by reducing mediator release from the mast cells.

1. Ephedrine is a weak sympathomimetic. Tolerance to the clinical effect can also develop.

2. Epinephrine (*Adrenalin*) induces $β_2$ effects.
  a. It also has α-agonistic effects that **reduce airway congestion**.
  b. Cardiovascular side effects, such as **increased blood pressure, heart rate, and myocardial contractility,** can be very pronounced.
  c. Epinephrine is the **treatment of choice for acute anaphylaxis.**

3. Isoproterenol (*Isuprel*) has much weaker actions on α-receptors than epinephrine and induces more vasodilation.
  a. **Increases in heart rate and contractility** can be very large, due to:
    (1) $β_1$ Effects on the heart
    (2) Reflexly mediated increases in sympathetic tone induced by the fall in blood pressure from the $β_2$-vasodilation.
  b. Repeated administration can result in an **anomalous bronchoconstriction.**
  c. The duration of action is **short** due to a rapid metabolism.

4. Terbutaline (*Bricanyl, Brethine*) and albuterol (*Proventil, Ventolin*) are relatively selective **$β_2$ agonists** with only weak effects on $β_1$ and α-receptors.
  a. A reflex-induced tachycardia will occur, due to the fall in blood pressure.
  b. A skeletal muscle tremor is the most common side effect.
  c. The non-catecholamine structure leads to a much **slower metabolism, a longer duration of action, and greater oral efficacy.**

D. The **glucocorticoids** are potent anti-inflammatory drugs that have the highest efficacy in the treatment of asthma.

1. They **reduce the inflammation** in the airways and enhance the $β_2$ effects of sympathetic activation on the airways.

2. Long term administration of the systemic glucocorticoids leads to **many side effects, including adrenal suppression, ulcers, and osteoporosis.**

3. Beclomethasone (*Beclovent, Vanceril*) is an **inhaled** glucocorticoid.
    a. Any drug that reaches the circulation is rapidly metabolized.
    b. The blood concentrations remain low and there are **fewer side effects** than with the systemic glucocorticoids.

E. Cromolyn (*Intal*) stabilizes mast cells, probably by reducing the calcium influx during mast cell degranulation.

    1. Mediator release is reduced.

    2. The onset of action is very slow, so it can only be used **for prophylaxis.**

F. Theophylline (*Slo-Bid, Theo-Dur*) **blocks adenosine receptors.** It also inhibits phosphodiesterases, which increases the concentration of cyclic adenosine monophosphate (cAMP); however, this does not occur at therapeutic concentrations.

    1. The rate of metabolism in the liver is quite variable between patients (e.g., smokers metabolize it faster than non-smokers).

    2. The side effects can be pronounced.
        a. CNS stimulation can progress to convulsions.
        b. Tachycardia and arrhythmias can occur.
        c. Rapid IV injections are dangerous due to marked cardiovascular effects.

    3. The blood theophylline concentrations should be monitored, because theophylline has a low therapeutic index.

G. Ipratropium (*Atrovent*) is an **inhaled quaternary anticholinergic.**

    1. Muscarinic blockade results in bronchodilation and reduced respiratory secretions.

    2. There are **no systemic anticholinergic effects** because it is not absorbed after inhalation.

H. Zafirlukast (*Accolate*), a **leukotriene antagonist,** and **zileuton** (*Zyflo*), a **lipoxygenase inhibitor,** are new drugs with potential value in the treatment of asthma.

VI. DRUGS FOR RHEUMATOID ARTHRITIS

A. Rheumatoid arthritis is an inflammatory disorder involving many organs in the body, including the joints.

B. Aspirin at high dosages has anti-inflammatory activity that reduces the symptoms of rheumatoid arthritis.

    1. The high dosages also saturate the metabolic enzymes and prolong the duration of action of aspirin.

    2. The most common side effects are **gastric irritation and GI bleeding.**

C. Other nonsteroidal anti-inflammatory drugs (NSAIDs), such as indomethacin (*Indocin*), tolmetin (*Tolectin*), ibuprofen (*Motrin*), sulindac (*Clinoril*) and naproxen (*Naprosyn*), also **act by inhibiting cyclooxygenase.**

    1. The side effects are **less pronounced** than with aspirin.
        a. All produce some **GI bleeding.**
        b. Renal toxicity may occur, as a reduction of prostaglandins in the kidney reduces renal blood flow and renal function. The resulting salt and water retention can reduce the effectiveness of most antihypertensives.
        c. Hepatitis can also be induced.

2. These drugs will decrease the pain and inflammation from arthritis, and the decreased inflammation can slow the joint damage. The disease continues to progress, however.

D. Antirheumatic drugs have **slow onsets** of action, taking months to induce an effect.

1. They have **no analgesic activity,** thus they should initially be combined with NSAIDs.

2. They **reduce the progression of joint erosion,** probably by reducing the phagocytosis and immune responses that are responsible for this autoimmune disease.

a. **Gold compounds** can be administered intramuscularly [e.g., **aurothioglucose** (*Solganal*)] or orally [e.g., **auranofin** (*Ridaura*)].

b. **Penicillamine** (*Cuprimine*), a chelator, can be given orally.

c. **Hydroxychloroquine** (*Plaquenil*), an antimalarial, is given orally; but can induce a **retinopathy.**

d. **Cyclophosphamide** (*Cytoxan*) has **cytotoxic** effects, such as bone marrow depression.

e. **Methotrexate** (*Rheumatrex*) is also a **cytotoxic** drug; however, it is effective at such low dosages that little toxicity actually occurs.

E. The glucocorticoids are the most potent anti-inflammatory drugs.

1. They have a fast onset of action.

2. Many side effects occur with chronic glucocorticoid administration, **including adrenal suppression, ulcers, and osteoporosis.**

3. Alternate day therapy may reduce the severity of these side effects.

4. Injection into a joint induces long term effects on the joint with little systemic toxicity.

F. Other rheumatoid and arthritic conditions are treated with the same groups of drugs, although the specific regimens may vary. The exception is gout.

VII. DRUGS FOR GOUT

A. A disorder of uric acid metabolism leads to the **hyperuricemia and acute gouty arthritis** that is characteristic of gout.

B. Many drugs can **reduce the gouty arthritic inflammation** without changing uric acid metabolism or elimination.

1. Colchicine may act by decreasing the release of chemotactic factors which attract leukocytes to the inflamed joints. This results in a reduction in the release of inflammatory mediators.

a. It has no effect on other inflammatory disorders, making it **useful in the diagnosis** of gout.

b. An **antimitotic** effect on the gastric mucosa frequently leads to a **bloody diarrhea.**

2. NSAIDs, such as indomethacin (*Indocin*), are very effective and safer than colchicine.

3. Glucocorticoids or adrenocorticotropic hormone (ACTH) will reduce the acute attack, but should not be used chronically due to their marked toxicity. Glucocorticoids can be given intra-articularly, if the arthritic pain is localized to one or a few joints.

C. Aspirin is contraindicated in patients with gout, because it can reduce the renal clearance of uric acid and increase the hyperuricemia.

D. The hyperuricemia can be reduced by 2 classes of drugs.

   1. **Uricosuric drugs,** such as **probenecid** (*Benemid*) and **sulfinpyrazone** (*Anturane*), **compete with uric acid transport** (especially reabsorption) in the proximal tubule of the kidney.

   a. The elimination of uric acid in the urine is increased.

   b. **Renal calculi** from uric acid crystals may form, thus the patient should ingest lots of **fluids with bicarbonate.**

   c. The mobilization of uric acid from the body stores **may induce an acute arthritic attack,** thus the patient should also be given colchicine or indomethacin.

   d. It is **inappropriate** to use uricosuric drugs:

   (1) During an **acute arthritic attack**

   (2) In patients with **renal failure**

   (3) When the **body burden of uric acid is very high,** such as in patients

   (a) With many tophi

   (b) With hematological disorders

   (c) During cancer chemotherapy

   2. **Inhibitors of uric acid synthesis** will reduce the production of uric acid, and are useful in patients who produce excessive amounts of uric acid.

   a. **Allopurinol** (*Zyloprim*) **inhibits xanthine oxidase.** It is also metabolized by xanthine oxidase to an active product, alloxanthine.

   (1) The uric acid concentration in the urine is reduced.

   (2) The **xanthine and hypoxanthine** concentrations in the urine are increased.

   (a) Xanthine and hypoxanthine are **more water soluble** than uric acid.

   (b) There are **multiple substances** in the urine, thus more total product can be excreted without causing crystalluria.

   b. The levels of 5-phosphoribosylpyrophosphate (PRPP), a precursor of purine synthesis, are also reduced by allopurinol.

   c. An acute attack can be induced, thus colchicine or indomethacin should be used in combination with the synthesis inhibitor.

VIII. DRUGS FOR ACNE

A. **Benzoyl peroxide** is a keratolytic that reduces acne.

B. Long-term treatment with **erythromycin or tetracyclines** is also effective.

C. **Isotretinoin** (*Accutane*), a vitamin A derivative, is administered orally for treatment of very severe cases of acne.

   1. It inhibits the sebaceous glands.

   2. The **side effects** can be very marked.

   a. It is **teratogenic.**

   b. **Hypervitaminosis A** can lead to irritated skin.

IX. VITAMINS

A. **Water-soluble vitamins are readily eliminated** by the kidney and are usually nontoxic.

B. **Fat-soluble vitamins can accumulate** and be more toxic, thus caution should be used if high doses are administered.

C. The deficiency and overdose syndromes for the vitamins are listed in Table 6–2.

Table 6–2

Deficiency and Toxic States for Vitamins

	Deficiency state	Toxic state
Water soluble vitamins:		
Thiamine (B$_1$)	Berberi (alcoholism)	
Riboflavin (B$_2$)	Infrequent	
Niacin (nicotinic acid, B$_3$)	Pellagra	$\downarrow$ serum triglycerides and cholesterol
		Flushing and GI distress
Pyridoxine (B$_6$)	Infrequent (isoniazid)	Peripheral neuropathy
		$\downarrow$ Anticonvulsant and L-dopa effects
Cyanocobalamin (B$_{12}$)	Pernicious anemia	
Folic acid	Anemia	
	Birth defects (anticonvulsants)	
Pantothenic acid	Infrequent	
Ascorbic acid (C)	Scurvy	
Biotin	Infrequent	
Fat soluble vitamins:		
Vitamin A	$\downarrow$ Dark adaptation	Dry, scaly skin
	Night blindness	
Vitamin D	Rickets	Hypercalcemia
Vitamin E	Infrequent	
Vitamin K	$\downarrow$ Blood coagulation	Jaundice in newborn
		$\downarrow$ Effect of oral anticoagulants

Drugs in parentheses can induce the deficiency states.
$\uparrow$ = increased; $\downarrow$ = decreased

D. The primary medical **uses** of vitamins are:

1. Treatment of **vitamin deficiencies**

2. **Prophylaxis** to avoid deficiencies in:
   a. Growing children
   b. Pregnant women
   c. Nursing mothers
   d. People on unusual diets

7

Endocrine Pharmacology

I. PITUITARY HORMONES

A. The release of **growth hormone** from the pituitary gland is regulated in an inhibitory fashion by the hypothalamic hormone somatostatin.

    1. Challenge tests are available to:

        a. Increase the release of growth hormone, including:

            (1) Insulin, which induces hypoglycemia

            (2) Bromocriptine

            (3) L-Dopa

        b. Decrease the release of growth hormone, including:

            (1) Glucose

            (2) Glucocorticoids, which induce hyperglycemia

            (3) Somatostatin

    2. **A growth hormone deficiency before puberty** will result in pituitary **dwarfism.**

        a. **Somatrem** (*Protropin*) and **somatropin** (*Humatrope*) are human grwoth hormone produced by recombinant DNA technology.

            (1) Replacement therapy will increase growth.

            (2) Replacement therapy is ineffective after epiphyseal closure has occurred in the long bones.

        b. **Androgens and estrogens** also increase growth; however, they are less effective than growth hormone, and can induce epiphyseal closure which limits further growth.

    3. **Excessive growth hormone** leads to **gigantism** before puberty and **acromegaly** after puberty.

        a. **Surgical removal** of part of the pituitary gland is the treatment of choice.

        b. **Bromocriptine** (*Parlodel*), a dopamine receptor agonist, inhibits growth hormone release in patients with excessive growth hormone. This is the opposite of the effect seen in normal subjects.

        c. **Octreotide** (*Sandostatin*), a somatostatin analogue, will also inhibit growth hormone release.

B. Deficiencies of **other important anterior pituitary hormones** can also lead to clinical symptoms.

    1. Challenge tests are available for these hormones.

        a. **Gonadotropin releasing hormone** (GnRH) should increase the serum levels of follicle stimulating hormone (FSH) and luteinizing hormone (LH).

        b. **Corticotropin releasing hormone** (CRH) should increase the serum levels of adrenal corticotropic hormone (ACTH).

    c. **Thyrotropin releasing hormone** (TRH) should increase the serum levels of thyroid stimulating hormone (TSH).

  2. The **end-organ hormones are used** for replacement therapy, rather than the pituitary hormones.

  3. The **glucocorticoids should be replaced before the thyroid hormones** to avoid adrenal insufficiency.

C The release of **vasopressin [antidiuretic hormone (ADH)]** from the **posterior pituitary** is important for the regulation of urine osmolarity. An inadequate vasopressin effect leads to **diabetes insipidus.**

  1. **Diagnosis** of the cause of the diabetes insipidus is based on the administration of vasopressin.

    a. If there is a **pituitary deficiency** of vasopressin, administered vasopressin will increase urine osmolarity.

    b. If the diabetes is **nephrogenic** in nature, administered vasopressin will have no effect on urine osmolarity.

  2. The **treatment** depends on the cause.

    a. If the diabetes insipidus is due to a **pituitary deficiency,** replacement therapy is instituted.

      (1) **Vasopressin** (*Pitressin*) can be given intramuscularly, but it can increase blood pressure.

      (2) **Lypressin** (*Diapid*), **administered intranasally,** has a duration of four hours.

      (3) **Desmopressin** (*DDAVP, Stimate*), administered intranasally, has a duration of **12 hours** and **does not increase blood pressure.**

    b. If the diabetes is **nephrogenic,** the **thiazides** (unexpectedly) are effective treatment.

D. **Oxytocin** (*Pitocin, Syntocinon*) is a posterior pituitary hormone that can be used to **increase uterine contractility.**

  1. **Estrogens increase and progestins decrease** the effects of oxytocin on the uterus.

  2. As term approaches, the number of oxytocin receptors in the uterine muscle increases; thereby increasing the sensitivity to oxytocin.

  3. The **primary use for oxytocin is to induce labor** at term.

    a. Low doses will increase the rhythmic contractions.

    b. High doses should be avoided because they can induce a sustained uterine contraction, leading to complications.

  4. **Ergonovine** (*Ergotrate*) also has oxytocic activity, however it induces a **sustained uterine contraction.** It is useful during the third stage of labor to:

    a. **Induce expulsion of the placenta**

    b. **Reduce postpartum hemorrhage** by compressing the uterine blood vessels

  5. **Premature labor** can be reduced by administering a β_2-**adrenoceptor agonist,** such as ritodrine (*Yutopar*).

II. ADRENOCORTICAL STEROIDS

A. **Cortisol,** also called hydrocortisone, is the primary adrenal glucocorticosteroid.

  1. **Transcortin [corticosteroid-binding globulin, (CBG)]** binds 75% of the cortisol in the circulation.

    a. Bound hormone is inactive.

     b. **Estrogens and thyroxine increase CBG,** but do not change the free cortisol concentration.

     c. **Androgens decrease CBG.**

2. Cortisol is metabolized by mixed function oxidases (MFOs) in the liver.

3. **The steroids diffuse** across the cell membranes and **bind to steroid receptors** in the cytoplasm. The steroid-receptor complex **migrates to the nucleus** and acts on DNA to **increase mRNA and protein synthesis.**

B. Three types of effects can be induced by these steroids.

    1. **Glucocorticoid effects** result from:
      a. **Enhanced gluconeogenesis** that leads to increased glucose production (diabetogenic) and increased glycogen synthesis and storage in the liver
      b. **Enhanced lipolytic effects** that redistribute fat

    2. **Mineralocorticoid effects** result from increased sodium ion exchange for potassium and hydrogen ions in the kidney.
      a. Hypokalemic alkalosis can be induced.
      b. The increased sodium load can lead to edema and hypertension.

    3. **Anti-inflammatory effects** occur, although the mechanism is not well established.

    4. The mineralocorticoid effects have been separated from the glucocorticoid and anti-inflammatory effects (Table 7–1). Dexamethasone is the most selective for glucocorticoid activity, and fludrocortisone is the most selective for mineralocorticoid activity. However, it has not been possible to separate the glucocorticoid actions from the anti-inflammatory actions.

C. There are **many side effects** that can occur with the adrenocorticoids, including:

    1. Hypokalemic alkalosis

    2. Glycosuria, which can aggravate diabetes mellitus

    3. Increased susceptibility to infections

    4. Peptic ulcers

    5. Myopathy

    6. Osteoporosis

    7. Symptoms of Cushing's syndrome

    8. Psychological effects

Table 7–1

Relative Mineralocorticoid to Glucocorticoid Activities of the Adrenocortical Steroids, As Compared to Cortisol (hydrocortisone)

Adrenocortical Steroid	Mineralocorticoid activity / Glucocorticoid activity
Cortisol [(hydrocortisone) (*Cortef, Cortril*)]	1
Cortisone (*Cortone*)	1
Prednisone (*Deltasone*)	0.1
Dexamethasone (*Decadron, Hexadrol*)	0.01
Fludrocortisone (*Florinef*)	10

9. ACTH suppression, which induces adrenal atrophy from which recovery takes several months. Thus withdrawal from long-term glucocorticoid treatment should be slow and tapered.

D. Several drugs can **inhibit adrenal** cortical function.

1. Aminoglutethimide (*Cytadren*) inhibits desmolase and reduces the production of all adrenal steroids.

2. Ketoconazole (*Nizoral*), an antifungal drug, reduces cortisol synthesis and release.

3. Spironolactone (*Aldactone*) inhibits aldosterone receptors.

E. There are many **clinical uses** for the adrenal steroids.

1. Adrenal insufficiency (Addison's disease) is treated with a glucocorticoid.

   a. Two thirds of the dose is administered in the morning to mimic the physiological levels.

   b. A mineralocorticoid is added if the insufficiency is primary (adrenal), but is usually not necessary for a secondary insufficiency (pituitary).

   c. For acute adrenal insufficiency, an intravenous glucocorticoid and saline are administered.

2. Congenital adrenal hyperplasia is due to an enzyme deficiency (e.g., 21-hydroxylase), which leads to increased ACTH release. It is treated with a glucocorticoid and a mineralocorticoid is added, if needed.

3. Dexamethasone is very useful in the **diagnosis** of Cushing's syndrome.

4. The anti-inflammatory effects of the adrenal steroids are very useful in the treatment of **allergic reactions, inflammatory diseases, tissue rejection, and leukemias.**

   a. They are safe during short-term therapy.

   b. Many side effects occur with long-term therapy.

      (1) It is possible to reduce the pituitary suppression, somewhat, by using **alternate-day therapy.** This involves doubling the dose one day and using only NSAIDs on the next day.

      (2) Adrenocortical steroids should be used for chronic therapy only as a last resort.

III. FEMALE SEX HORMONES

A. Sex hormone binding globulin binds estradiol and testosterone.

B. Effects of estrogens include:

1. Control of reproductive organs

2. Control of sex characteristics

3. Anabolic effects that promote growth, which are less than with androgens

C. The **estrogen preparations** are:

1. Estradiol (*Estrace*), which is usually conjugated (*Premarin*) for a longer duration of action.

2. Ethinyl estradiol (*Estinyl*)

3. Mestranol

4. Diethylstilbestrol (*Stilphostrol*), which is **non-steroidal**

D. Effects of the **progestins** include:

1. Induction of the **secretory changes in the endometrium of the uterus** that are necessary for pregnancy

2. Induction of **menstruation,** when the progestin levels fall.

E. The **progestin preparations** are:

1. Progesterone, which is not useful due to a very short half-life

2. Medroxyprogesterone (*Provera*)

3. Norethindrone (*Norlutin*), which has some androgenic activity

4. Levonorgestrel (*Norplant*)

F. Side effects have been ascribed mostly to the estrogens.

1. Some have **minor** consequences, such as
  a. Nausea and vomiting
  b. Edema
  c. Breast tenderness

2. Some have **major** consequences, such as
  a. **Thrombophlebitis, deep vein thrombosis, and pulmonary embolism.** The increased risk is similar to the risk during pregnancy.
  b. **Breast cancer** (controversial) and **endometrial cancer**
  c. Fluid retention and mild hypertension

G. There are many **uses** for the female sex steroids.

1. **Contraceptives** can act by many different mechanisms.
  a. **The combined oral estrogen-progestin** (from days 5 to 25) **reduces FSH and LH release** by the negative feedback inhibitory action of the estrogen on the pituitary, and this reduces ovulation. The new preparations have lower estrogen concentrations to reduce the side effects.
  b. **The continuous oral progestins (minipills)** reduce implantation of the fertilized ovum.
  c. Depot medroxyprogesterone (*Depo-Provera*) or levonorgestrel (*Norplant*) are progestins that are useful when compliance is a concern.
  d. **Acute, high-dose estrogen therapy** is used, postcoitally, to reduce implantation.
  e. The gonadotropin releasing hormone agonists, which are **really partial agonists** that reduce FSH and LH release, are being tested as contraceptives.
  f. **Mifepristone (RU 486) is an anti-progesterone** substance that blocks the preparation of the uterus for pregnancy. It is usually combined with prostaglandins when used to induce abortions.
  g. Nonoxynol-9 acts as a spermicide.
  h. The sequential estrogen (days 5 to 25) and progestin (days 20 to 25) oral contraceptives were withdrawn from the market because they induce endometrial cancer.

2. **Hypogonadism** is treated by replacement therapy with physiological doses of sex steroids.
  a. **Menopausal symptoms** are induced by the loss of female sex hormones.
    (1) **Estrogens will decrease the symptoms of menopause.**
    (2) Estrogens will **decrease the risk of osteoporosis and heart disease.**
    (3) **Progestins** are usually added to the regimen to reduce the high incidence of **endometrial cancer** when estrogens are used alone.
  b. **Amenorrhea** can also be treated with sex hormones.
    (1) Estrogen–progestin preparations will **induce menstruation.**
    (2) **Growth and sexual development** will be induced when the sex hormones are administered at the age of puberty.

    c. **Dysfunctional uterine bleeding** can be treated with sex hormones.

  3. **Inhibition of ovarian function** can be induced by pharmacological doses of sex steroids.

    a. **Dysmenorrhea** is reduced, due to the inhibition of ovulation. Indomethacin is also effective because it inhibits prostaglandin release, which may be involved in inducing the dysmenorrhea.

    b. **Hirsutism** due to ovarian androgens is reduced.

    c. **Postpartum lactation** is suppressed.

    d. **Some cancers** are treatable with sex hormones or sex hormone antagonists.

H. An inappropriate indication for estrogens is a threatened miscarriage. If used in such a manner, estrogens can induce **vaginal adenomas in female offspring after puberty,** and may also affect male offspring.

IV. FERTILITY DRUGS

A. **Clomiphene** (*Clomid*) is an **antiestrogen that reduces the feedback inhibition** of estrogen on the pituitary gland and hypothalamus.

  1. Increased release of FSH and LH **enhances ovulation.**

  2. A functional pituitary gland and functional ovaries are required.

  3. The incidence of multiple pregnancies is increased.

B. **Human menopausal gonadotropins** (hMG) (*Pergonal*) and **human chorionic gonadotropins** (hCG) (*Follutein, Pregnyl*) have **FSH and LH activities;** thus a functional pituitary gland is not required.

C. **GnRH** preparations act on the pituitary gland.

  1. Pulsatile administration of **gonadorelin** (*Factrel*) induces the release of FSH and LH.

  2. Sustained administration of **leuprolide** (*Lupron*) decreases the release of FSH and LH, which is useful in the **treatment of infertility from endometriosis.**

D. **Danazol** (*Danocrine*) is a testosterone derivative that reduces gonadotropin release.

  1. Endometrial atrophy is produced, which reduces **endometriosis.**

  2. Upon discontinuing the danazol, fertility is increased.

E. **Bromocriptine** (*Parlodel*) is a **dopamine receptor agonist** that reduces prolactin release from the pituitary gland. It increases fertility in patients with **hyperprolactinemia.**

V. MALE SEX HORMONES

A. These sex hormones have **androgenic and anabolic** activities.

B. Many **preparations** are available.

  1. **Testosterone** is usually administered, **intramuscularly,** as an ester (*Delatestryl*) to prolong the duration of action.

  2. **Methyltestosterone** (*Metandren, Testred*) and **fluoxymesterone** (*Halotestin*) are effective when given **orally** and have longer durations of action than testosterone.

  3. **Nandrolone** (*Durabolin*) is an **anabolic** steroid, although it still has some androgenic effects.

C. The **side effects** include:

1. Masculinization

2. Edema

D. The **uses** for the male sex hormones include:

1. Treatment of hypogonadism
   a. Potency and fertility (if given with gonadotropins) are increased.
   b. Growth is increased, although epiphyseal closure induced by the steroids can limit further growth.

2. Treatment of cryptorchism, for which **hCG** is used

3. Treatment of prostate cancer, for which leuprolide (*Lupron*) is used

4. Anabolic actions
   a. To hasten recovery after an injury
   b. To treat anemias

E. An inappropriate use of the steroids is to increase athletic performance. The anabolic steroids can cause:

1. Reduced growth, after an initial growth spurt, by inducing **premature epiphyseal closure** in young athletes

2. Reduced fertility due to feedback inhibition by the steroids on gonadotropin release

3. Virilization in females

4. Hepatotoxicity and hepatic tumors

5. Edema and hypertension

F. Spironolactone (*Aldactone*) and **flutamide** (*Eulexin*) have **antiandrogen activity** and can be used to treat hirsutism, prostate cancer, and precocious puberty.

VI. THYROID HORMONES

A. The thyroid preparations include:

1. Levothyroxine (T_4) (*Levothroid, Synthroid*), which is a pure chemical
   a. It is **highly bound** to thyroxine binding globulin (**TBG**).
   b. The half-life is **7 days.**

2. Liothyronine (**L-triiodothyronine,** T_3) (*Cytomel*), which is also **a pure chemical**
   a. It is less well bound than T_4 to TBG, thus it is **more potent.**
   b. The half-life is **1 day,** which is much shorter than the half-life of T_4.

3. Desiccated thyroid, which is powdered animal thyroid glands

4. Thyroglobulin (*Proloid*), which is extracted from animal thyroids

5. Liotrix, which is a combination of T_4 and T_3

6. TSH (*Thytropar*) and **TRH (protirelin)** (*Thypinone*), which are used for diagnostic purposes

B. Hypothyroidism, whether primary, secondary, or tertiary in nature, is the major indication for the thyroid hormone preparations.

1. T_4 is usually preferred, and treatment is initiated slowly to avoid **cardiovascular** symptoms.

2. T_4 will reduce the symptoms of hypothyroidism and reduce TSH release which reduces the goiter.

3. T_3 has too rapid an onset, and is only preferred for the treatment of hypothyroid coma.

4. **Side effects** from hormone replacement are due to an **increase in metabolic rate** and include:
   a. **Flushing**
   b. **Weight loss**
   c. **Increased appetite**
   d. **Tachycardia**
   e. **Angina**

5. In the hypothyroid newborn, aggressive treatment within one month of birth is necessary to avoid cretinism. After 3–4 months of untreated hypothyroidism in the newborn, brain dysfunction will occur.

C. **Antithyroid drugs** act by several different mechanisms.

   1. **The thioamides,** such as **propylthiouracil and methimazole** (*Tapazole*) inhibit thyroid hormone synthesis.
      a. **Reduced I_2 binding to tyrosine and reduced coupling of iodotyrosines** leads to a depletion of thyroid hormones.
         (1) The release of T_4 and T_3 is reduced.
         (2) Increased TSH release from reduced feedback inhibition can induce a **goiter.**
         (3) The onset is very **slow** because the large stores of hormones have to be depleted.
      b. Propylthiouracil also inhibits the peripheral conversion of T_4 to T_3.

   2. **Iodide in large amounts** rapidly reduces thyroid hormone release, although the effect is transient. It also reduces the vascularity of the thyroid gland.

   3. **Radioactive iodine (^{131}I)** is concentrated in the thyroid, where β-irradiation can destroy some of the thyroid cells.

   4. **Thiocyanate and perchlorate** block the iodide concentrating mechanism in the thyroid. They are not used, however, because aplastic anemia can be induced.

   5. **The sympathetic blockers** [e.g., propranolol (*Inderal*)] do not affect the thyroid, but do rapidly **reduce the myocardial stimulation** that occurs with elevated thyroid hormone levels.

D. **Hyperthyroidism** can be treated in three ways.

   1. Administration of **thioamides** will reduce the synthesis and release of thyroid hormones.
      a. Since a goiter can occur if the patient becomes hypothyroid, T_4 may be added to the regimen to reduce TSH release.
      b. This is not a permanent cure.
      c. Propylthiouracil and methimazole do cross the placenta and will affect the fetus.

   2. **A partial thyroidectomy** can result in a permanent cure.
      a. Possible adverse consequences of surgery are hypoparathyroidism and **hypothyroidism.**
      b. Propylthiouracil or iodide are used pre-operatively to reduce the size and vascularity of the thyroid gland.

> **3.** ^{131}I, given orally, will destroy some of the thyroid cells. ^{131}I treatment:
>> **a.** Has a **slow onset**
>> **b.** Can result in **hypothyroidism**
>> **c.** **Must be avoided during pregnancy**
>> **d.** Could theoretically induce genetic abnormalities (but probably doesn't)

> **E.** **Thyroid storm** (acute hyperthyroid crisis) can be treated with **propranolol and antithyroid drugs.**

> **F.** **Thyroid cancer** can be treated with ^{131}I, if the cancer cells concentrate iodide.

VII. HORMONES AFFECTING CALCIUM METABOLISM

> **A.** Three hormones are involved in the regulation of the serum calcium concentration (Figure 7–1).

>> **1.** **Parathyroid hormone** release, induced by hypocalcemia, increases serum calcium by increasing the:
>>> **a.** **Formation of active 1,25 dihydroxyvitamin D_3 in the kidney**
>>> **b.** **Absorption of calcium in the gut**
>>> **c.** **Bone resorption of calcium**
>>> **d.** **Kidney reabsorption of calcium** (and increasing phosphate excretion)

>> **2.** **Vitamin D_3** from the diet or from exposure to sunlight is hydroxylated to **25 hydroxyvitamin D_3, calcifediol** (*Calderol*), in the liver.
>>> **a.** This intermediate is further hydroxylated in the kidney to **1,25 dihydroxyvitamin D_3, calcitriol** (*Rocaltrol*).

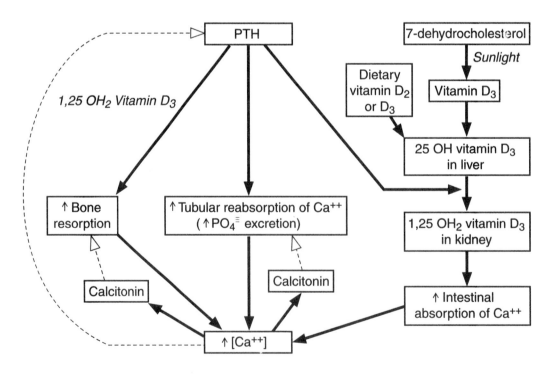

Figure 7–1. Regulation of calcium metabolism by parathyroid hormone, vitamine D and calcitonin. Ca^{++} = calcium; OH = hydroxy; OH_2 = dihydroxy; $PO_4^{=}$ = phosphate; PTH = parathyroid hormone

     b. Dihydroxyvitamin D_3 **increases the intestinal absorption of calcium.**

   3. **Calcitonin** release, in response to hypercalcemia, decreases bone resorption.

B. **Hypoparathyroidism** results in hypocalcemia, hyperphosphatemia and increased membrane excitability (hypocalcemic tetany).

   1. **Treatment** involves the administration of a **vitamin D preparation and calcium.** Parathyroid hormone is not very useful as it must be given intramuscularly.

   2. **Calcitriol is preferred for acute treatment.**

   3. **Pseudohypoparathyroidism** can be treated with high doses of vitamin D, which appear to directly increase bone resorption.

C. **Osteomalacia** (hypovitaminosis D) is also treated with a **vitamin D preparation.**

   1. If GI absorption is poor, vitamin D can be administered parenterally.

   2. If liver function is reduced, calcifediol or calcitriol can be administered.

   3. If kidney function is reduced, calcitriol or **dihydrotachysterol** (*Hytakerol*) can be administered.
      a. Dihydrotachysterol has a **rapid onset.**
      b. It is metabolized in the **liver** to the active form.

D. **Hyperparathyroidism** results in **hypercalcemia.**

   1. **Surgery** is the preferred mode of treatment.

   2. **Corticosteroids** can be used to **reduce the absorption of calcium** by the intestine.

   3. **Acute treatment** involves the administration of:
      a. **Fluids**
      b. **Loop diuretics,** which increase calcium excretion by the kidneys
      c. **Phosphate,** if hypophosphatemia is present

E. **Hypervitaminosis D** results in hypercalcemia and is acutely treated much like hyperparathyroidism.

F. **Osteoporosis** is a skeletal disorder in which calcium hormone function is normal.

   1. **Treatment of postmenopausal osteoporosis involves the administration of:**
      a. **Vitamin D**
      b. **Calcium**
      c. **Estrogen**
         (1) Estrogens reduce bone resorption, but apparently do not restore lost bone.
         (2) **Progestins** are given to reduce the risk of endometrial cancer.
         (3) **Raloxifene** (*Evista*) is a selective estrogen receptor modulator which:
            (a) Stimulates bone and lowers serum lipids.
            (b) Has no effect on the endometrium or breasts.

   2. **Other treatment modalities** can be used.
      a. **Calcitonin** can be administered, intranasally.
      b. **Alendronate** (*Fosamax*) is a phosphonate that stabilizes bone.

G. **Paget's disease** involves a rapid turnover of the calcium in bone. **Treatment** utilizes:

   1. **Calcitonin** (*Calcimar*), parenterally. Salmon calcitonin is the most active form.

   2. **Etidronate** (*Didronel*), which is a phosphonate that reduces bone turnover. It is **effective when given orally** and has the same efficacy as calcitonin.

VIII. DRUGS FOR DIABETES MELLITUS

A. Diabetes is caused by an inadequate effect of insulin that can lead to **hyperglycemia, ketonemia,** and **ketoacidosis.**

B. Type 1 (insulin-dependent) diabetes mellitus results from the loss of endogenous insulin, while type 2 (non-insulin-dependent) diabetes mellitus is probably due to insulin resistance.

C. There are many **preparations** with hypoglycemic actions.

    1. **Insulin** is a **polypeptide** that is ineffective when given orally and is usually administered intramuscularly or subcutaneously.

        a. Several sources are available.

            (1) **Bovine insulin** has three amino acids that are different from human insulin.

            (2) **Porcine insulin** has only one amino acid that is different from human insulin. It is available as a conventional or a purified (less antigenic) preparation.

            (3) **Human insulin** (*Humulin*) is produced by recombinant DNA technology.

        b. **Regular insulin (crystalline zinc insulin)** has a fast onset and is the only insulin preparation that can be given intravenously. It also has a short duration of action.

        c. Insulin is conjugated with proteins or crystallized in various forms which slows the onset and increases the duration of action. **NPH** and **lente insulins** with durations up to 24 hours are the most useful.

        d. **Lispro insulin** (*Humalog*) is a new rapid acting, short duration preparation.

    2. **Oral antidiabetic drugs** are also available.

        a. **The sulfonylureas increase the insulin release** from the pancreas, and enhance the peripheral effectiveness of insulin, thus a functional pancreas is required.

            (1) **Tolbutamide** (*Orinase*) is short acting and is metabolized in the liver by oxidation.

            (2) **Chlorpropamide** (*Diabinese*) is long acting and is partially excreted in the unchanged form by the kidney.

            (3) **Glyburide** (*DiaBeta, Micronase*) and **glipizide** (*Glucotrol*) are second generation sulfonylureas.

        b. **Metformin** (*Glucophage*) is a biguanide that **enhances the hepatic response** to insulin.

        c. **Acarbose** (*Precose*) is an **α-glucosidase inhibitor** which slows the breakdown of carbohydrates in the gut.

        d. **Troglitazone** (*Rezulin*) **reduces insulin resistance** in type 2 diabetes mellitus.

D. **The side effects** of insulin and the sulfonylureas can be very severe.

    1. **Hypoglycemia** can occur from excessive doses, inadequate food intake, exercise, or alcohol.

        a. **CNS effects,** which can progress to convulsions, lead to a **sympathetic activation** (e.g., tachycardia). Propranolol will block this sympathetic activation making it more difficult for diabetics to sense that they are hypoglycemic.

        b. The hypoglycemia can be **reversed by:**

            (1) Ingestion of candy, orange juice, or other **sugar** source

            (2) **Glucagon, intramuscularly or subcutaneously**

            (3) **Glucose, intravenously**

2. **Insulin antibodies** can lead to **resistance** to insulin. The risk of antibody formation for the insulin preparations is: bovine > porcine > purified porcine > human.

3. Increases in body weight frequently occur.

E. **Treatment** of diabetes involves **balancing of caloric intake, exercise, and hypoglycemic medications.**

    1. The diet is a major factor in diabetic control, and the caloric intake should be constant and regular.

    2. Patients with **type 1** diabetes mellitus must use **insulin.**

    3. Patients with **type 2** diabetes mellitus can use either **insulin** or **oral hypoglycemic drugs.** Insulin is preferred for type 2 diabetes mellitus in patients with:
      a. Reduced renal function
      b. Reduced hepatic function
      c. Gestational diabetes
      d. Persistent hyperglycemia
      e. Cardiovascular risk factors

    4. The efficacy of treatment should be followed by **self-monitoring of blood glucose** by the patient.

    5. Effective treatment should **nearly eliminate the acute symptoms** of diabetes, including the hyperglycemia, glycosuria, polyphagia, polydipsia, polyuria, hypoglycemia, and ketoacidosis.

    6. Based on clinical studies, **rigid control** of blood glucose **probably also reduces the chronic complications** of diabetes, including:
      a. **Neuropathy**
      b. **Retinopathy**
      c. **Nephropathy**
      d. **Cardiovascular disease**

F. **Diabetic ketoacidosis or hyperosmolar (non-ketotic) coma** should be managed with:

    1. **Fluid and electrolytes, especially potassium**

    2. Crystalline zinc insulin, intravenously

    3. Correction of acidosis

    4. Carbohydrates

IX. DRUGS FOR HYPOGLYCEMIA

A. **Glucagon,** which is physiologically released from alpha cells in the pancreas, **increases glycogenolysis and gluconeogenesis.**

    1. These actions **increase the blood glucose** concentration in diabetics who are hypoglycemic.

    2. The effectiveness will be lost when the **glycogen stores are depleted.**

    3. It is a polypeptide that must be given **parenterally.**

B. **Glucose** can be administered orally or parenterally to treat hypoglycemia in diabetics.

C. **Diazoxide** (*Proglycem*) is an antihypertensive, when given intravenously.

    1. After **oral** administration, it **reduces insulin release** from the pancreas; thus it is ineffective for the treatment of insulin-induced hypoglycemia.

    2. It is useful to treat the hypoglycemia from a **hyperinsulinoma.**

D. Many hormones can increase the serum glucose concentration, including:

    1. Glucocorticoids

    2. Growth hormone

    3. Epinephrine

    4. Estrogens and progestins

    5. Thyroid hormone

8
Drugs for Bacterial Infections

I. PRINCIPLES OF BACTERIAL CHEMOTHERAPY

A. Bacterial chemotherapy involves the administration of drugs that **kill or slow the growth of bacteria without affecting host cells.** This phenomena is called **selective toxicity.**

B. **Bactericidal drugs kill bacteria,** often by inhibiting cell wall synthesis.

    1. Bactericidal drugs include
        a. β-Lactams
            (1) Penicillins
            (2) Cephalosporins
            (3) Aztreonam
            (4) Imipenem
        b. Aminoglycosides
        c. Quinolones
        d. Vancomycin

    2. Bactericidal drugs are necessary for
        a. Patients with severe infections
        b. Patients with severe or debilitating diseases
        c. Patients who are immunocompromised

C. **Bacteriostatic drugs** only **inhibit replication of bacteria,** often by reducing protein synthesis.

    1. The immune system eradicates the infection.

    2. Bacteriostatic drugs include:
        a. Tetracyclines
        b. Erythromycin
        c. Chloramphenicol
        d. Clindamycin
        e. Sulfonamides
        f. Trimethoprim

D. **Single drugs are preferred** to treat infectious diseases, unless a drug combination is the accepted mode of therapy (usually to reduce the development of resistance). Inappropriate drug combinations can:

    1. Increase the incidence of side effects

    2. Result in antagonism between drugs

    3. Increase the risk of superinfections

E. **Bacterial resistance to drugs** can be

    1. **Natural** (e.g., no target site in the bacteria)

    2. **Acquired**

        a. Resistance acquired by **mutation** is unusual, although it is common with tuberculosis (TB) because there is a large population of bacteria (See XIV "Drugs for Tuberculosis").

        b. Resistance acquired by **R-factors** on plasmids is a common, **very rapid** method of acquiring resistance that often involves resistance to many antibiotics.

F. **Superinfections** due to an **overgrowth of insensitive indigenous microbes,** such as *Pseudomonas, Clostridium,* and *Candida,* are most prevalent

    1. With broad-spectrum antibiotics

    2. With long-term therapy

    3. In patients with severe illnesses

G. Changes of the bacterial flora in the gastrointestinal tract that are induced by antibiotics frequently lead to symptoms of GI irritation, such as nausea, vomiting, and diarrhea.

II. PENICILLINS

A. The **active nucleus** of the penicillin molecule is a 4-membered ring, called the **β–lactam ring** (Figure 8–1).

B. Penicillin binds to **penicillin binding proteins** and induces many effects that inhibit cell wall synthesis (e.g., **inhibition of transpeptidases**).

    1. **Cross-linking of the bacterial cell wall is reduced.**

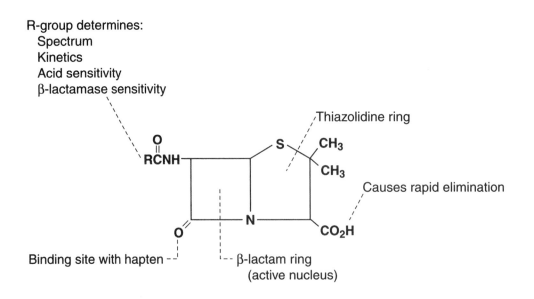

Figure 8–1. The general structure of the penicillins

2. The cell wall is weakened and the bacteria rupture due to the high internal osmotic pressure, thus the penicillins are **bactericidal.**

C. The **pharmacokinetics** of penicillin G affect how it is used.

   1. It is relatively **unstable in acid,** thus the bioavailability is low. It can be administered orally, however, the serum penicillin concentrations are variable after this route of administration.

   2. There is **poor penetration into the cerebrospinal fluid (CSF),** unless inflammation is present.

   3. **Active renal tubular secretion** results in a short half-life.
      a. Probenecid, which blocks the active secretion, will reduce the renal clearance of penicillin G.
      b. Procaine penicillin G, intramuscularly, and benzathine penicillin G, intramuscularly, have long durations of action due to slow absorption from the site of injection.

D. Although the penicillins are very safe antibiotics, they have some important **adverse effects.**

   1. **Hypersensitivity** reactions can develop.
      a. **Immediate hypersensitivity** reactions, characterized by **anaphylaxis,** occur within 20 minutes.
         (1) Penicillin interacts with proteins to form **minor determinants** which act as haptens for inducing the immediate hypersensitivity reaction.
         (2) The reaction is mediated by **IgE antibodies.**
      b. **Accelerated** (occurring within 1 day) and **delayed** (occurring within 1 week) reactions are less severe.
         (1) Penicilloic acid, which is a product of the breakdown of penicillins, interacts with proteins to form the **major determinants,** which act as haptens for inducing the reactions.
         (2) These reactions are mediated by **IgG or IgM antibodies.**
      c. Patients may display hypersensitivity to the first dose. This hypersensitivity is probably due to the environmental levels (e.g., in food) of penicillins.
      d. **Cross-sensitivity between the penicillins** is very high.
      e. **Skin tests** are available to check for hypersensitivity.
         (1) Penicillin G is somewhat unreliable.
         (2) Penicilloyl-polylysine is a major determinant.
         (3) Minor determinants are not widely available.
      f. **Anaphylactic reactions** should be treated with **epinephrine.**

   2. **Superinfections** can develop, especially with the broad-spectrum penicillins, such as ampicillin.

   3. **Sodium loading** from the penicillins is most common with carbenicillin and ticarcillin, which are disodium salts.

   4. **Convulsions,** caused by γ-aminobutyric acid (GABA) receptor blockade, can be induced at high dosages of penicillins.

   5. **Non-allergic skin rashes** can occur with ampicillin, especially in patients with infectious mononucleosis.

E. The **spectrum** of penicillin G includes:

   1. **Gram-positive bacteria**

   2. **Gram-negative cocci,** but not most other gram-negative bacteria

F. Resistance to penicillin G is due to **penicillinases or β-lactamases,** which split the active part of the molecule, the β-lactam ring.

G. Amidases are used to alter the side chain of penicillin G (Table 8–1), resulting in groups of:

   1. Natural penicillins. Penicillin V is more effective after oral administration than penicillin G.

   2. Penicillinase-resistant penicillins. These penicillins are useful for the treatment of infections involving penicillinase-producing bacteria.

   3. Extended-spectrum penicillins. These penicillins have more gram-negative activity than penicillin G.

H. All extended-spectrum penicillins are penicillinase-sensitive.

   1. Either **clavulanic acid** or **sulbactam,** which are **β-lactamase inhibitors,** may be combined with the extended-spectrum penicillins.

   2. Resistant organisms will be more sensitive to this combination.

III. CEPHALOSPORINS

A. The structure of the cephalosporins (Figure 8–2), with a β-lactam ring and a dihydrothiazine ring, is very similar to that of the penicillins.

   1. The pharmacological **properties** are also similar to those of the penicillins.

   a. Inhibition of transpeptidases leads to an inhibition of cell wall synthesis resulting in a **bactericidal** effect.

   b. Most cephalosporins are eliminated by active tubular secretion in the kidney.

   c. Penetration into the CSF is poor, unless inflammation is present.

   d. The **side effects** are also similar to those from the penicillins.

   (1) Hypersensitivity can occur.

   (a) There is **some cross-hypersensitivity with the penicillins.**

   (b) In patients with a history of a mild accelerated or mild delayed reaction to a penicillin, the cephalosporins may be considered.

Table 8–1
Properties of the Penicillins

	Effectiveness when taken orally	Resistance to penicillinases	Spectrum
Natural penicillins			
Penicillin G	Variable	None	Narrow
Penicillin V (*Pen-Vee, V-Cillin*)	Good	None	Narrow
Penicillinase-resistant penicillins			
Methicillin (*Staphcillin*)	Poor	Yes	Narrow
(side effect: nephritis)			
Cloxacillin (*Tegopen, Cloxapen*)	Good	Yes	Narrow
Nafcillin (*Unipen*)	Variable	Yes	Narrow
Dicloxacillin (*Dynapen*)	Good	Yes	Narrow
Extended-spectrum penicillins			
Ampicillin (*Omnipen*)	Good	None	Broad
(side effect: non-allergic rash)			
Amoxicillin (*Amoxil, Larotid*)	Better	None	Broad
Carbenicillin (*Geocillin*)	Very active against *Pseudomonas & Proteus*		
Ticarcillin (*Ticar*)	Very active against *Pseudomonas & Proteus*		

R$_1$-group determines:
  Spectrum
  β-lactamase sensitivity

Figure 8–2.   The general structure of the cephalosporins

        (c) In patients with a history of an immediate reaction to a penicillin, the cephalosporins should be avoided.
    (2) **Superinfections** can occur.
    (3) **Nephrotoxicity** has been reported.

2. The cephalosporins also have important **differences from the penicillins.**
    a. The anti-bacterial **spectrum is broader.**
    b. They are **more resistant to β-lactamases.**
    c. Only a few are effective when taken orally.

3. Three generations of cephalosporins are available.
    a. **First-generation** cephalosporins include cefazolin (*Ancef,Kefzol*) and oral cephalexin (*Keflex*).
        (1) These have **narrow spectrums for cephalosporins,** but the spectrums are similar to ampicillin.
        (2) They have some resistance to β-lactamases.
        (3) They are the **most active** cephalosporins **for gram-positive bacterial infections.**
    b. **Second-generation** cephalosporins include cefoxitin (*Mefoxin*), oral cefuroxime (*Zinacef*), and oral cefaclor (*Ceclor*). They have broader spectrums and more resistance to β-lactamases.
    c. As a group, the **third-generation** cephalosporins have:
        (1) The **broadest spectrums**
        (2) The **highest activities against gram-negative bacteria**
        (3) The **lowest activities against gram-positive bacteria**
        (4) The **highest resistance to β-lactamases**
        (5) The **highest lipid solubilities**
        (6) The **best penetration into the CSF**
    d. There are also some unique properties of **individual third-generation cephalosporins.**

(1) Ceftriaxone (*Rocephin*) has the **longest half-life** (8 hours) of any cephalosporin.

(2) Cefixime (*Suprax*) is an **oral** preparation.

(3) Ceftazidime (*Fortaz*) is the best **anti-pseudomonal** cephalosporin.

(4) Cefoperazone (*Cefobid*) is eliminated **(70%) in the bile,** and is thus very useful in patients with renal failure.

IV. OTHER β-LACTAMS

A. Aztreonam (*Azactam*) is a **monobactam.**

1. It decreases cell wall formation, and thus is **bactericidal.**

2. Only **aerobic gram-negative bacteria,** especially *Pseudomonas*, are affected. There is no activity against gram-positive bacteria or anaerobes.

3. It is resistant to most β-lactamases.

4. The kinetics are similar to the penicillins, although it must be **administered parenterally.**

B. **Imipenem with cilastatin** (*Primaxin*) inhibits cell wall transpeptidation.

1. This results in **bactericidal** activity against most bacteria, thus imipenem has a **very broad spectrum.**

2. It is resistant to most β-lactamases.

3. It **distributes to most tissues** in the body.

4. Imipenem is **nephrotoxic.**
   a. Metabolism of imipenem in the kidney by **dehydropeptidases** leads to an inactive product that is nephrotoxic.
   b. **Cilastatin inhibits the dehydropeptidases** and eliminates the nephrotoxicity, thus it is always administered in combination with imipenem.

V. AMINOGLYCOSIDES AND SPECTINOMYCIN

A. Aminoglycosides

1. Representatives of this class of antibiotics include **gentamicin** (*Garamycin*), **tobramycin** (*Nebcin*), **amikacin** (*Amikin*), neomycin (*Mycifradin*) and streptomycin.

2. **Inhibition of protein synthesis** occurs as a result of **irreversible** aminoglycoside binding to the **30S ribosomal subunit.**
   a. An inactive initiation complex is formed.
   b. Misreading of the mRNA template occurs.

3. Although aminoglycosides act as protein synthesis inhibitors, they are **bactericidal.** This may be due to the irreversible binding at the site of action.

4. The **selective toxicity** may relate to the fact that **humans do not have the 30S ribosomal subunits.**
   a. Mammals have 80S ribosomes composed of 60S and 40S subunits.
   b. Bacteria have 70S ribosomes composed of 50S and 30S subunits.

5. Aminoglycosides are only active against **gram-negative bacteria** that are **aerobes,** because the drugs must be accumulated in the bacteria by active transport, which is oxygen-dependent. The activity is maintained even after the plasma drug concentration falls. This is called a **post-antibiotic effect.**

6. The **pharmacokinetics** are typical for large, polar molecules.

      a. **Parenteral administration** is necessary.

      b. Distribution is limited to the extracellular fluid.

      c. They **do not reach the CSF.**

      d. **Elimination** occurs via **glomerular filtration,** thus the creatinine clearance is used to determine the maintenance dose.

   7. **Resistance** is mediated by **R-factors** transmitted by conjugation.

      a. Bacterial **enzymes** can inactivate the aminoglycosides.

      b. Membrane uptake of the aminoglycosides can be reduced.

      c. Amikacin induces a much lower incidence of microbial resistance than the other aminoglycosides.

   8. The aminoglycosides are **very toxic.**

      a. **Ototoxicity** can lead to:

        (1) **Loss of equilibrium**

        (2) **Loss of hearing**

      b. **Nephrotoxicity** can occur.

      c. **Neuromuscular blockade** can reduce respiratory function, especially after surgery.

   9. An aminoglycoside in combination with a β-lactam provides broad (empiric) antibiotic treatment.

B. Spectinomycin (*Trobicin*) also **inhibits protein synthesis** by binding the 30S ribosomal subunit.

   1. It is only **bacteriostatic.**

   2. The only important indication is as an alternate treatment for **gonorrhea.**

VI. TETRACYCLINES

A. This class of antibiotics includes **tetracycline** (*Achromycin, Panmycin*) and **doxycycline** (*Vibramycin*), which are **bacteriostatic inhibitors of protein synthesis.**

   1. Reversible binding to the **30S ribosomal subunit** inhibits the acceptor (A) site on the mRNA.

   2. Binding of tRNA to the mRNA-ribosomal complex is blocked.

B. **Selective toxicity** occurs because the tetracyclines are **actively accumulated by bacteria,** but not actively accumulated by host cells.

C. **Resistance** is mediated by **R-factors** that **reduce the active drug accumulation.**

D. The **pharmacokinetics** vary depending on the specific drug.

   1. All tetracyclines are administered orally. Tetracycline, in particular, is **chelated and inactivated by calcium (milk), magnesium, aluminum (antacids) and iron,** and should be taken when the stomach is empty. Doxycycline is less avidly chelated and can be taken with a meal.

   2. Some tetracyclines are cleared by metabolism in the liver and some are cleared by glomerular filtration in the kidney.

   3. **Doxycycline,** uniquely, is cleared as a **chelate in the feces.** The elimination is not dependent on either liver or kidney function.

E. The **spectrum is very broad,** and the tetracyclines are especially useful for infectious diseases involving *Chlamydia, Rickettsia,* and *Mycoplasma.*

F. These antibiotics have few **side effects.**

1. Do not administer tetracyclines to children because chelation of calcium
   a. Can **discolor developing teeth**
   b. Can **reduce growth** in developing bone

2. Photosensitivity can occur.

3. Hepatotoxicity and nephrotoxicity have been reported.

4. As they have broad spectrums, **superinfections** from *Clostridium* and *Candida* can develop.

VII. ERYTHROMYCIN

A. This **macrolide** antibiotic is a **bacteriostatic** inhibitor of protein synthesis. Reversible binding to the **50S** ribosomal subunit of gram-positive microorganisms inhibits translocation of the peptidyl molecule from the A-site to the P-site on the mRNA.

B. It is effective when taken orally and is **eliminated in the bile** in the unaltered form.

C. Reduction of mixed function oxidase (MFO) activity enhances the effects of many drugs metabolized by MFOs (e.g., theophylline).

D. The spectrum is limited to **gram-positive bacteria.**

   1. Erythromycin (*Ilosone, Erythrocin*) is especially useful for infectious diseases involving *Chlamydia*, *Mycoplasma* and *Legionella*.

   2. It is also a useful alternative to the penicillins for gram-positive infections.

E. Cholestatic hepatitis can occur as a side effect.

F. New macrolides have been introduced.

   1. Clarithromycin (*Biaxin*) is **more stable in acid** than erythromycin.

   2. Azithromycin (*Zithromax*) has a **long half-life** (3 days).

VIII. CHLORAMPHENICOL

A. Bacteriostatic inhibition of protein synthesis results from reversible binding of chloramphenicol (*Chloromycetin*) to the **50S** ribosomal subunit.

   1. This decreases the binding of tRNA to the A–site.

   2. As a result, protein elongation is reduced.

B. It is effective when **given orally, penetrates membranes very well,** and **readily reaches the CSF.**

C. Metabolism by glucuronyl transferase **(glucuronide conjugation)** occurs in the liver.

D. Toxicity is a major limitation with chloramphenicol.

   1. A **gray baby syndrome** can be induced when chloramphenicol is administered to newborns. **Slow metabolism,** which is due to a lack of glucuronyl transferase, results in toxic blood concentrations of chloramphenicol when standard doses are administered.

   2. Anemias can be induced.
      a. Dose-dependent bone marrow depression results from inhibition of mitochondrial 70S ribosomes.
      b. An infrequent, **irreversible aplastic anemia** that is **not dose-related** and is **frequently fatal** has limited the usefulness of chloramphenicol to seriously ill patients who cannot be treated with safer drugs.

E. The **spectrum** of activity is **very broad, including anaerobes,** but it is only used as an alternative drug to treat infections, such as *Salmonella typhi* and *Haemophilus influenzae*. It is bactericidal for *H. influenzae*.

F. **Resistance** occurs due to **R-factors** that code for the enzyme, chloramphenicol **acetyltransferase,** which acetylates and inactivates the drug.

IX. CLINDAMYCIN

A. **Bacteriostatic inhibition of protein synthesis** results from binding of clindamycin (*Cleocin*) to the 50S ribosomal subunit.

B. Clindamycin is effective when given **orally** and is useful to treat **anaerobic infections,** such as *Bacteroides*.

C. The incidence of **pseudomembranous colitis** (a superinfection from *Clostridium difficile*) is high and this limits the usefulness of clindamycin. This superinfection should be **treated with metronidazole** or vancomycin, given orally.

X. VANCOMYCIN

A. **Binding of vancomycin** (*Vancocin*) **to cell wall precursors** leads to an **inhibition of cell wall synthesis** that is **bactericidal.**

B. Because it is poorly absorbed by the oral route, vancomycin is given **intravenously** except when being used to treat enteric infections.

C. It is cleared by renal **glomerular filtration.**

D. The high activity of vancomycin against **gram-positive microorganisms** makes it useful as the last alternative to treat **methicillin-resistant *Staphylococcus aureus*.**

E. **Side effects** include:

   1. Ototoxicity

   2. Nephrotoxicity

   3. Erythema ("red neck syndrome"), due to histamine release

XI. QUINOLONES

A. **Norfloxacin** (*Noroxin*) and **ciprofloxacin** (*Cipro*) inhibit bacterial **DNA gyrases,** which results in a **bactericidal** effect. They are structurally similar to nalidixic acid, a urinary tract antiseptic.

B. **Resistance** develops due to a mutational **change in the gyrase.**

C. The **spectrum** is **very broad,** although there is **no effect on anaerobes.**

D. Both oral and intravenous administration are effective, and the drugs distribute widely in the body.

E. **Elimination** is due to **renal secretion** of the active drug.

F. Erosion of cartilage by the quinolones can lead to tendinitis and tendon rupture.

XII. SULFONAMIDES AND TRIMETHOPRIM

A. The sulfonamides [e.g., sulfisoxazole (*Gantrisin*)] are **analogues of para-aminobenzoic acid (PABA)** that compete with PABA in the synthesis of folic acid (Figure 8–3).

   1. The **decrease of tetrahydrofolic acid** inhibits DNA synthesis, primarily by decreasing thymidylate synthesis.

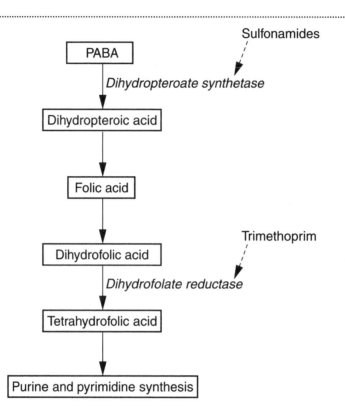

Figure 8–3.   The synthesis of folic acid. The sites of sulfonamide and trimethoprim actions are indicated. PABA=para-aminobenzoic acid

2. **Selective toxicity** occurs because:
   a. **Bacteria have no active transport for folate and must synthesize it.** This synthesis is blocked by the sulfonamides.
   b. **Humans cannot synthesize folate.** They must obtain it from the diet and it is actively transported into the host cells. Inhibition of folate synthesis has no host effects.

3. These drugs are usually **bacteriostatic;** although with the selective absence of thymine, they can be bactericidal.

4. The **spectrum is very broad** and they **distribute to all body fluids.**

5. The major limitation of the sulfonamides is the **R–factor mediated resistance** which is very common.

6. **Side effects** can usually be avoided.
   a. **Displacement of bilirubin** from plasma albumin binding sites can induce **kernicterus** in the newborn.
   b. Due to their poor solubility, some of the older sulfonamides can **crystallize in the urine.**
   c. **Hypersensitivity reactions** (e.g., Stevens-Johnson syndrome) do occur, particularly with the long-acting sulfonamides which are now rarely used.
   d. **Hemolytic anemia** can be induced.

7. The important **indications** for use of the sulfonamides are:
   a. Urinary tract infections that are acute and uncomplicated
   b. Recurrent otitis media

B. Trimethoprim (*Proloprim, Trimpex*) is a **competitive inhibitor of dihydrofolate reductase.**

   1. This inhibitory action leads to effects on folic acid synthesis that are similar to the sulfonamides, although the onset is more rapid.

   2. Selective toxicity occurs because the **bacterial reductase is 20,000 times as sensitive** as the human reductase.

C. Trimethoprim and the **sulfonamides** (e.g., sulfamethoxazole) are usually combined (*Bactrim, Septra*).

   1. A **synergistic** effect occurs with the combination because 2 steps in folic acid synthesis are inhibited.

   2. This is a very useful combination for treating:
   a. Recurrent urinary tract infections
   b. Chronic prostatitis
   c. Nocardiosis
   d. *Pneumocystis carinii*
   e. Upper respiratory tract infections from *Haemophilus influenzae*

   3. The combination can induce a **folate deficiency in the host,** leading to an **anemia** that is treatable with folinic acid.

XIII. MISCELLANEOUS ANTIMICROBIALS

A. Urinary tract antiseptics are rapidly eliminated in the active form by the kidney, so the drug concentrations in the urine are very high. This makes them useful for treating urinary tract infections.

   1. Nitrofurantoin (*Macrodantin*) damages DNA and has a **broad antimicrobial spectrum.**

   2. Methenamine (*Mandelamine*) is broken down by the **low pH** of urine to **formaldehyde,** which is bactericidal, especially against **gram-negative bacteria.**

B. Bacitracin (*Baciguent*) inhibits cell wall synthesis by **decreasing precursor transport** to the cell wall.

C. Polymixin B and **colistin** (*Coly-Mycin*) **increase membrane permeability,** leading to the loss of essential intracellular substances.

XIV. DRUGS FOR TUBERCULOSIS

A. Drug combinations, often initially with 4 drugs, are always used in the long-term treatment (9–12 months) of TB to **avoid the development of antibiotic resistance.** Single drug therapy is only useful for preventive purposes.

B. Isoniazid (*Nydrazid*) alters the **synthesis of mycolic acid,** which is a cell wall component in the *Mycobacterium.*

   1. It is **bactericidal,** although resistance develops rapidly by mutation due to the large population of bacteria in an active infection.

   2. Oral administration of isoniazid is effective and the drug **distributes to all body fluids** and to all sites of infection.

3. Clearance from the body involves **acetylation** in the liver, the rate of which has a **genetic** variation.

   a. Fast acetylators will have lower blood concentrations.

   b. Slow acetylators are more likely to develop toxicity.

   c. The rate of metabolism is reduced by phenytoin or carbamazepine.

4. Side effects from isoniazid include:

   a. **Hepatitis,** which increases in incidence with **age**

   b. **Peripheral neuritis** due to increased pyridoxine excretion. This can be avoided by giving **pyridoxine.**

C. **Rifampin** (*Rifadin, Rimactane*) inhibits the β-subunit of DNA-dependent RNA **polymerase,** which reduces RNA synthesis in the bacteria.

   1. Rifampin is also **bactericidal** for *Mycobacterium* and has **good penetration** into tissues and tuberculous lesions.

   2. It is also used **prophylactically** for patients exposed to:

      a. *Neisseria meningitidis*

      b. *Haemophilus influenzae,* type b

   3. **Metabolism** in the liver results in a metabolite that is eliminated in the bile. It does activate MFOs.

   4. Side effects include:

      a. **Hepatotoxicity**

      b. **Orange coloring of tears, sweat, and urine**

      c. **A flu-like syndrome**

D. **Pyrazinamide** is **bactericidal** and effective when given orally.

E. **Ethambutol** (*Myambutol*) inhibits mycolic acid synthesis, but is only **bacteriostatic.** It can also **impair red–green vision.**

F. **Streptomycin** is **bactericidal,** but it must be administered **parenterally,** does not penetrate into cells, and **does not distribute** as widely in the body as the other drugs.

G. Treatment of **leprosy** (*Mycobacterium leprae*) involves drug combinations of:

   1. **Sulfones** [e.g., **dapsone** (*Alvosulfon*)] which are PABA analogues that reduce folic acid synthesis.

   2. Rifampin

   3. Thalidomide (*Thalomid*)

9

Drugs for Infections from Eukaryotic Organisms and Viruses

I. ANTIFUNGAL DRUGS

A. Amphotericin B (*Fungizone*) **binds ergosterol** in fungal cells and **increases the membrane permeability** by forming membrane pores.

    1. Amphotericin B is **fungicidal** at high dosages.
        a. It is the drug of choice for most systemic fungal infections.
        b. It has no antibacterial activity.

    2. Selective toxicity occurs because there is less binding to cholesterol in host cell membranes.

    3. **Slow parenteral** administration is necessary.

    4. The **side effects** are **very severe,** including:
        a. A **febrile response**
        b. A **delayed nephrotoxicity**

B. Flucytosine (*Ancobon*) is metabolized by deaminases in the fungal cells to the active substance, **fluorouracil.**

    1. Fluorouracil inhibits fungal DNA and RNA synthesis.

    2. An advantage of flucytosine is **wide distribution,** even to the CNS.

C. Ketoconazole (*Nizoral*) interferes with **ergosterol synthesis,** thereby increasing fungal membrane permeability.

    1. It is only **fungistatic;** but it can be administered **orally.** The bioavailability is reduced if the gastric pH is high (e.g., with antacids).

    2. It is a valuable alternative to amphotericin because of its effectiveness when administered orally and its mild side effects.
        a. **Hepatotoxicity** can occur.
        b. **Inhibition of MFOs** will slow the metabolism of many drugs. Cortisol and testosterone synthesis can also be reduced.

D. Fluconazole (*Diflucan*) has properties that are similar to ketoconazole, except:

    1. Intestinal absorption of the drug is **not affected by changes of gastric pH**

    2. It can be given **intravenously**

    3. Penetration to the CSF is better

E. Nystatin (*Nilstat, Mycostatin*) acts like amphotericin B in that it binds ergosterol; however, it is only used **topically.**

F. **Griseofulvin** (*Gris-PEG, Grisactin*) **binds to keratin** in skin, hair, and nails.

    1. **Disruption of mitotic spindles,** which decreases mitosis, leads to a fungistatic action.

    2. Griseofulvin has a **very low water solubility.**

        a. The duration of action is very long (months) after oral administration.

        b. It undergoes metabolism in the liver and activates the MFOs.

II. ANTIPROTOZOAL DRUGS

A. **Malaria** is a common protozoal disease in tropical climates.

    1. **Blood schizonticidal drugs** clear the *Plasmodium* from the erythrocytes.

        a. **Chloroquine** (*Aralen*) is selectively **concentrated** ($100\times$) by red blood cells that are infected with the parasites.

            (1) It acts on all erythrocytic *Plasmodium* infections, **except chloroquine-resistant *Plasmodium falciparum.***

            (2) **Once a week, oral administration** is effective because chloroquine is highly concentrated in the liver and has a long half-life.

        b. **Pyrimethamine** (*Daraprim*) **inhibits dihydrofolate reductase,** leading to reduced folic acid synthesis, especially in parasites.

            (1) It is often combined with a sulfonamide [(e.g., sulfadoxine (*Fansidar*)].

            (2) **Teratogenicity** has been reported in animals.

        c. **Quinine** has a **very rapid onset** and short duration, making it useful for treating a **severe acute attack. Side effects** are:

            (1) **Cinchonism**

            (2) **Arrhythmias**

        d. **Mefloquine** (*Lariam*) is a quinine derivative that has a **long half-life** and can be administered orally.

        e. Tetracyclines also have some antimalarial activity.

    2. **Primaquine** is the only drug which can eliminate the tissue forms of the parasites.

        a. It is active on the **exoerythrocytic forms** and the gametes of *Plasmodium vivax* and *Plasmodium ovale*.

        b. **Hemolytic anemia** can occur in patients with a glucose-6-P-dehydrogenase deficiency.

    3. **Prophylaxis** is usually provided for travelers to countries where malaria is endemic.

        a. **Chloroquine or mefloquine** (1 dose/week) is given from 1 week before the trip to 4 weeks after.

        b. **Primaquine** may be added during the last 2 weeks, although this has become controversial due to primaquine toxicity.

B. **Amebiasis** involves both gastrointestinal and tissue sites.

    1. **Metronidazole** (*Flagyl*) acts on *Entamoeba histolytica* in the intestinal and hepatic sites, but does not eliminate the intestinal cysts.

        a. It **inhibits anaerobic metabolism** in *Entamoeba, Gardnerella, Bacteroides,* and *Clostridium*.

        b. A **disulfiram-like** reaction can occur, if alcohol is ingested.

    2. **Iodoquinol** (*Yodoxin*) is an **intestinal amebicide** that is not absorbed, thus there are no systemic effects or side effects.

    3. **Dehydroemetine** acts primarily on the extraintestinal forms, but it can produce cardiac toxicity.

C. Other infections respond to drug therapy.

    1. *Toxoplasma gondii* infections are treated with pyrimethamine and a sulfonamide.

2. *Pneumocystis carinii* infections are treated with trimethoprim and sulfamethoxazole.

3. Metronidazole is useful to treat infections from:
   a. *Trichomonas vaginalis*
   b. *Giardia lamblia*

III. ANTHELMINTICS

A. Anthelmintics are used to treat parasitic worm infections due to cestodes, nematodes, or trematodes.

B. **Cestode** infections (*Taenia saginata, Taenia solium, Diphyllobothrium latum* and *Hymenolepis nana*) can be treated with **praziquantel** (*Biltricide*).

   1. **Muscle stimulation and paralysis** are induced in the helminths.

   2. **Vacuolization of the cuticle** also occurs.

   3. The tissue forms of *T. solium* (cysticercosis) are also effectively treated.

C. The specific treatment of a nematode infection will depend on the type of nematode involved.

   1. **Intestinal nematodes** (*Enterobius, Ascaris, Trichuris, Necator,* and *Ancylostoma*) are the easiest to treat because the drugs do not have to be absorbed into the body of the host.
      a. **Pyrantel** (*Antiminth*) **activates nicotinic cholinoceptors** inducing a **muscle paralysis** in the helminth.
      b. **Mebendazole** (*Vermox*) **inhibits glucose uptake.**
      c. **Albendazole** (*Zentel*) is also effective.

   2. **Tissue nematodes** can be divided into 2 types.
      a. **Filarial nematodes** include *Wuchereria, Brugia, Onchocerca, Loa,* and *Dipetalonema.*
         (1) **Diethylcarbamazine** (*Hetrazan*) may increase the helminth susceptibility to the host **immune system.**
            (a) It is **most active against the microfilaria** and least active against the adult filaria.
            (b) An **allergic reaction** can result from the parasitic break-down products.
         (2) **Ivermectin** (*Mectizan*) **opens GABA-sensitive chloride channels** which induces a muscle paralysis.
      b. **Non-filarial tissue nematodes** include *Angiostrongylus* and *Trichinosis.*
         (1) **Thiabendazole** (*Mintezol*) **inhibits fumarate reductase,** which is unique to helminths.
         (2) **Mebendazole** (*Vermox*) and **albendazole** (*Zentel*) are also effective.

D. **Trematode** infections, such as schistosomiasis, can be treated with **praziquantel** (*Biltricide*).

IV. ANTIVIRAL DRUGS

A. **Amantadine** (*Symmetrel*) and **rimantadine** (*Flumadine*) act on RNA viruses by **inhibiting the uncoating** of viral nucleic acids, which reduces viral replication.

   1. These drugs are used primarily for the **prophylaxis** of **type A influenza viral infections.**

   2. **Treatment** with either of these drugs is effective if initiated **within 48 hours** after the initial appearance of symptoms.

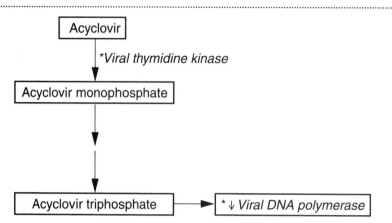

Figure 9–1. Mechanisms of selective toxicity (*) for acyclovir.

B. Acyclovir (*Zovirax*) is a guanine analogue that is a relatively safe antiviral drug.

   1. It is safe because it has **2 sites** of selective toxicity (Figure 9–1).

   a. **Only viruses can phosphorylate acyclovir to acyclovir monophosphate.**

   b. **Acyclovir triphosphate is more active on viral DNA polymerases.**

   2. The clinical **indications** include:

   a. **Genital and labial herpes simplex virus (HSV) types 1 or 2. There is no effect on the latent forms.**

   b. **Herpes encephalitis and keratitis**

   c. **Varicella-zoster virus**

C. **Ganciclovir** (*Cytovene*) is an analogue of acyclovir that is used for **cytomegalovirus (CMV) and Epstein-Barr virus** infections.

D. **Foscarnet** (*Foscavir*) is an alternate drug for the treatment of **mucocutaneous HSV and CMV.**

E. **Idoxuridine** (*Herplex*) is a thymidine analogue.

   1. The triphosphate form is incorporated into viral DNA, which leads to a reduction of viral protein synthesis.

   2. It is used for topical treatment of herpes simplex infections of the eye.

F. **Ribavirin** (*Virazole*) is used to treat the **respiratory syncytial virus.**

G. **Zidovudine** (*Retrovir*), formerly called azidothymidine (AZT), is a thymidine analogue that is converted to the triphosphate form, which is then incorporated into viral DNA and terminates viral DNA synthesis.

   1. Zidovudine **inhibits HIV reverse transcriptase.**

   2. It is used in the treatment of **HIV-positive and AIDS patients.**

   3. **Bone marrow depression** may occur.

H. **Didanosine** (*Videx*) is another reverse transcriptase inhibitor that is used in HIV patients.

I. **Ritonavir** (*Norvir*) acts by **inhibiting proteases** that cleave viral protein precursors. It is used in combination with drugs like AZT and didanosine for the treatment of HIV.

10

Cancer Chemotherapy

I. PRINCIPLES OF CANCER CHEMOTHERAPY

A. Most anticancer drugs **affect cell division.**

1. They act preferentially on **rapidly proliferating cells.**

2. **Smaller tumors have a higher growth fraction.**
   a. Consequently, they are more susceptible to the anticancer drugs.
   b. **Adjuvant chemotherapy** is used with surgery or radiation to treat undetectable metastases, when they are small and highly sensitive to anticancer drugs.

3. Cells in phase G_0 **(non-dividing) will survive** chemotherapy.

B. Some drugs are **cell cycle phase specific.**

1. **Methotrexate** kills in **S-phase** (DNA synthesis phase).

2. **Vincristine and vinblastine** kill in **M-phase** (mitotic phase).

C. **Cells are killed in a first-order manner** (a constant percentage is killed with each course of therapy).

D. Immunocompromised patients usually respond less well to anticancer treatment.

E. **Combination therapy** is common.

1. Each drug in the combination should be **active** against the tumor.

2. The drugs should have **different mechanisms** of action.

3. The drugs should have **different toxicities.**

4. Time must be allowed for host tissue recovery between treatment cycles.

F. There are many **standard toxicities** that occur with most anticancer drugs.

1. **Myelosuppression** is common because the bone marrow is a rapidly proliferating tissue.
   a. This is usually the dose-limiting side effect.
   b. The leukopenia is greater than the thrombocytopenia, which is greater than the anemia.
   c. The drugs for which bone marrow depression is not the dose–limiting toxicity include:
   (1) Hormones
   (2) Vincristine
   (3) Bleomycin

(4) Asparaginase
(5) Cisplatin

2. **Other rapidly proliferating cells** that are affected include:
   a. GI epithelium
   b. Germinal epithelium
   c. Hair follicles

3. **Nausea and vomiting** are common side effects and can be managed with:
   a. Phenothiazines
   b. Dronabinol (*Marinol*)
   c. Metoclopramide (*Reglan*)
   d. Ondansetron (*Zofran*)

4. **Tissue necrosis** may occur at the site of injection.

5. Some anticancer drugs have **unique organ toxicities.**
   a. Daunorubicin and doxorubicin are cardiotoxic.
   b. Bleomycin induces pulmonary toxicity.
   c. Vincristine is neurotoxic.
   d. Cisplatin is nephrotoxic.

6. **Mutagenicity, teratogenicity and carcinogenicity** can occur, especially with the alkylating agents.

7. **A large cell kill** can lead to **hyperuricemia** and crystalluria. These can be reduced with **allopurinol** (*Zyloprim*).

II. ANTICANCER DRUGS

A. Alkylating agents are usually cell cycle **phase non-specific.**

1. **Nitrogen mustards** form a very reactive **immonium** intermediate.
   a. The intermediate attacks nucleophilic groups, especially **guanine,** leading to:
      (1) Cross-linking of DNA
      (2) Linking of bases in the same DNA strand
      (3) Linking of bases to water or other molecules
   b. Compounds with **2 reactive sites** have **greater activity.**
   c. The cells will not replicate normally.
   d. The cells can repair the DNA; thus, the mustards are **proliferation dependent** because rapidly dividing cells have less time to repair the DNA before DNA replication occurs.
   e. Resistance occurs due to:
      (1) Reduced drug uptake by the cancer cells
      (2) Increased rate of DNA repair
   f. Cross-resistance between alkylating agents is common.
   g. Bone marrow depression is the dose-limiting side effect for these drugs.
   h. Many nitrogen mustards are available.
      (1) Mechlorethamine (*Mustargen*) is a potent **vesicant** with a **very short half-life** (a few minutes).
         (a) It reacts with tissues quickly, especially those near the site of injection.
         (b) Phlebitis occurs at the injection site.
      (2) Cyclophosphamide (*Cytoxan*) is a **prodrug** which is metabolized to active products.
         (a) Hydroxycyclophosphamide and phosphoramide mustard are 2 active alkylating metabolites.

(b) As the prodrug form is inactive, it can be given **orally** and it is not a vesicant.

(c) The metabolites are eliminated in the urine which can irritate the bladder, leading to a **sterile hemorrhagic cystitis.**

(3) **Chlorambucil** (*Leukeran*), effective after oral administration, is the slowest-acting alkylating agent and the least toxic.

(4) **Melphalan** (*Alkeran*) acts similarly.

2. Several **nitrosoureas** have alkylating effects.

   a. **Lomustine** (*CCNU, CeeNu*) and **carmustine** (*BiCNU*) are **highly lipophilic.**

   (1) They can **penetrate to the CSF.**

   (2) Unlike most other cytotoxic drugs, they are useful to treat CNS cancers or metastases in the CNS.

   b. **Streptozocin** (*Zanosar*) accumulates in the **beta cells of the pancreas** and can produce **insulin shock,** which is an unusual side effect for an anticancer drug.

3. **Busulfan** (*Myleran*), **thiotepa** (*Thioplex*), and **dacarbazine** (*DTIC*) are other alkylating anticancer drugs.

4. **Cisplatin** (*Platinol*) is an alkylating agent that binds to guanine in the DNA molecule.

   a. It is not phase-specific.

   b. **Nephrotoxicity** is the dose-limiting side effect.

B. **Antimetabolites** are usually **phase-specific, especially S-phase–specific.**

1. **Methotrexate** (*Folex*)is an analogue of folic acid which competitively inhibits the enzyme, **dihydrofolate reductase.**

   a. Tetrahydrofolate levels are decreased.

   (1) Decreased DNA, RNA and protein synthesis occurs.

   (2) The primary effect is a decrease of **thymidylate synthesis.**

   (3) The highest activity occurs with low thymidine derivatives and normal RNA and normal proteins.

   b. It is S–phase specific and **self–limited** because it slows the movement of cells into the S–phase.

   c. Toxicity can be **reversed by leucovorin** (citrovorum factor) which is directly converted to tetrahydrofolate.

   d. Resistance can be due to:

   (1) Increased production of dihydrofolate reductase

   (2) Decreased affinity of the enzyme for methotrexate

   (3) Decreased active transport of methotrexate into the cancer cells

   e. Due to a low water solubility, **crystalluria and renal damage** can occur.

2. **Purine analogues** must be phosphorylated to be active.

   a. **Thioguanine** is converted to thioguanine monophosphate and deoxythioguanosine triphosphate, which is **incorporated into tumor cell DNA.**

   (1) Thioguanine monophosphate also inhibits amidotransferases, which leads to reduced purine synthesis.

   (2) It is G_1 and S-phase specific.

   (3) Resistance is usually due to increased drug inactivation.

   b. **Mercaptopurine** (*Purinethol*) is converted to thioinosine monophosphate, which inhibits amidotransferase.

   (1) It is **inactivated by xanthine oxidase.**

   (2) As a result, **allopurinol** will decrease the metabolism and increase the toxicity of mercaptopurine.

3. Fluorouracil (*Efudex, Adrucil*) is an important **pyrimidine analogue.**
  a. The phosphorylated form, fluorodeoxyuridine monophosphate, decreases the activity of thymidylate synthase.
  b. This effect can be enhanced by leucovorin and reversed by thymidine.
  c. It is S-phase specific.

C. Some **antibiotics** can be used as anticancer drugs.

  1. **Dactinomycin** (*Cosmegen*), also called actinomycin D, **intercalates** between bases, especially guanine, in DNA.
   a. This reduces DNA-dependent RNA polymerase activity, which reduces RNA synthesis.
   b. It is cytotoxic at **all phases** of the cell cycle and is **not proliferation dependent.**
   c. Resistance occurs due to decreased drug entry into the cells.

  2. **Doxorubicin** (*Adriamycin*) and **daunorubicin** (*Cerubidine*) also **intercalate** into DNA, but there is **no base specificity.**
   a. Resistance occurs due to decreased drug entry into the cells and there is cross-resistance between doxorubicin and daunorubicin, and often with dactinomycin.
   b. A **cumulative cardiotoxicity** occurs due to **superoxide anion.**

  3. **Bleomycin** (*Blenoxane*) induces **fragmentation of DNA.**
   a. The effects of intercalating agents are enhanced.
   b. **Delayed pulmonary toxicity** can be produced.

D. **Steroid hormones** can produce palliation of some cancers.

  1. Their activity depends on the presence of the **steroid receptors** (e.g., estrogen receptors).

  2. Hormone active substances include the antiestrogen tamoxifen (*Nolvadex*), estrogens, progestins, androgens, and corticosteroids.

E. There are several **inhibitors of chromosomal function.**

  1. The vinca alkaloids, **vincristine** (*Oncovin*) and **vinblastine** (*Velban*), enhance the **depolymerization** of the **tubulin in the mitotic spindles,** thereby disrupting spindle function.
   a. **Mitosis is inhibited (M-phase specific).**
   b. Vinblastine displays standard toxicity, however **neurotoxicity is the dose-limiting side effect of vincristine.**

  2. **Etoposide** (*VePesid*) **inhibits topoisomerases,** resulting in breaks of the DNA strands. Cells are arrested in late S- or G_2-phase.

  3. **Paclitaxel** (*Taxol*) **enhances microtubule formation** and thereby affects cell division.

F. **Miscellaneous drugs** have unique actions.

  1. **Asparaginase** (*Elspar*) metabolizes asparagine and glutamine.
   a. Tumors with no asparagine synthetase are sensitive to asparaginase, because any asparagine taken up by the tumors will be metabolized.
   b. It has none of the standard anticancer drug toxicities.
   c. **Hypersensitivity** reactions can occur due to the proteinaceous nature of this drug.

  2. **Mitotane** (*Lysodren*) induces an adrenocortical necrosis and is useful to treat adrenocortical cancers.

III. IMMUNOMODULATORS

A. Immunosuppressants are used to suppress the rejection of transplanted organs.

    1. **Corticosteroids** act on many processes to suppress the immune response.

        a. They have **no cytotoxic activity.**

        b. **Anti-inflammatory** effects are very useful.

    2. **Cytotoxic drugs suppress the bone marrow,** and thereby reduce the immune reaction. They have **no anti-inflammatory effects.**

        a. **Azathioprine** (*Imuran*) is a **purine analogue** which reduces DNA synthesis.

            (1) It is **S-phase specific.**

            (2) The side effect profile is similar to the anticancer drugs.

        b. **Cyclophosphamide** (*Cytoxan, Neosar*) is a **phase non-specific** immunosuppressant.

        c. **Methotrexate** (*Folex*) is also useful.

    3. **Cyclosporine** (*Sandimmune*) is a **selective immunosuppressant.**

        a. **T-lymphocyte activation is reduced,** probably as a result of decreased interleukin release.

        b. B-lymphocyte and mature T-lymphocyte functions are not affected.

        c. There is **no myelosuppression.**

        d. **Nephrotoxicity** is the major complication.

B. The immune potentiator, **levamisole** (*Ergamisol*), increases the proliferation of T-lymphocytes. It is useful in a combination regimen to treat colon cancer.

11

Toxicology

I. EMERGENCY TOXICOLOGY

A. The **goals of treatment** of a patient who has been exposed to a toxic substance are (in sequential order):

1. Control the symptoms, including
- **a.** Cardiovascular changes
- **b.** Loss of respiratory function
- **c.** Convulsions
- **d.** Acidosis

2. Reduce the absorption of the substance

3. Administer an antidote

4. Enhance the elimination of the substance

B. Several approaches are available to **reduce the systemic absorption of an ingested toxic substance.**

1. Emesis can be induced.
- **a.** Agents
  - **(1)** Syrup of ipecac acts as a local irritant on the gastrointestinal (GI) tract and stimulates the chemoreceptor trigger zone (CTZ) in the CNS to induce vomiting.
    - **(a)** It is sold without a prescription.
    - **(b)** It should be administered as soon as possible, and less than 4 hours after ingestion, to maximize the recovery of the toxic substance.
  - **(2)** Apomorphine is much less useful as an emetic, because
    - **(a)** Parenteral administration is required.
    - **(b)** Respiratory depression, as with other narcotics, can occur.
- **b.** Emesis has several **contraindications,** including:
  - **(1)** Ingestion of a **strong acid or alkali**
  - **(2)** Ingestion of a **low viscosity petroleum distillate** (e.g., kerosene), which could be aspirated during emesis
  - **(3)** An **unconscious** patient
- **c.** The primary **complication** of emesis is **aspiration** of the stomach contents, which can lead to pneumonitis.

2. Gastric lavage (pumping the stomach) is also effective.
- **a.** Lavage should be performed **as soon as possible.**
- **b.** The **contraindications are the same** as for emesis, except it can be performed in a comatose patient.
- **c.** **Aspiration of the stomach contents** can also occur with this method.

3. Chemical adsorption with activated charcoal can be utilized after emesis or lavage.
  a. Charcoal binds many, but not all, toxic substances.
  b. One limitation is that charcoal will also bind emetics, antidotes, and dietary substances.

4. Water can be used to dilute a toxic substance, especially strong acids and bases.

5. Osmotic cathartics will reduce the absorption by enhancing the elimination of a toxic substance in the feces, but this is often ineffective.

C. Elimination of toxic substances from the circulation **can occasionally be hastened.**

  1. The rate of **metabolism** of a toxic substance usually cannot be affected, although the hepatotoxicity of acetaminophen can be reduced by this mechanism.
    a. With an **overdose of acetaminophen,** glutathione will be depleted. This results in the build-up of a reactive intermediate that induces a **delayed hepatotoxicity.**
    b. Acetylcysteine, administered shortly after exposure to acetaminophen, will replenish the glutathione, enhance the conjugation of the reactive acetaminophen intermediate, and reduce the hepatotoxicity.

  2. The **urinary excretion** of a toxic substance can occasionally be enhanced.
    a. Osmotic or loop diuretics will increase urine flow and enhance clearance of a toxic substance by the kidney.
    b. Changing the pH of the urine will enhance the elimination of some toxic substances by ion trapping (converting the substance to the charged form, which cannot be reabsorbed across the nephron wall).
      (1) To be effective, the pK_a of the toxic substance should be **near 7.5** and the V_d must be small.
      (2) Bicarbonate enhances the elimination of the **salicylates and phenobarbital** (weak acids).
      (3) Ammonium chloride enhances the elimination of **phencyclidine and amphetamines** (weak bases).

  3. Hemodialysis or peritoneal **dialysis** can be effective if the toxin:
    a. Is a small molecule and readily crosses membranes
    b. Has a small V_d, so much of the substance is in the serum
    c. Has low protein binding, so much of the substance is in the free form.

  4. Hemoperfusion can also be performed.

II. HEAVY METAL TOXICITY AND CHELATORS

  A. Chelators are substances that bind heavy metals. When heavy metals have been absorbed, chelators are administered for therapeutic purposes. A metal-chelate complex is formed, which is then **excreted.**

    1. Dimercaprol (*BAL*) chelates arsenic, mercury, gold, and lead. It must be administered **parenterally.**

    2. Penicillamine (*Cuprimine, Depen*) chelates arsenic, mercury, gold, lead, and copper.
      a. It can be administered **orally.**
      b. A penicillin allergy can develop.
      c. Wilson's disease is an indication for use.

    3. Deferoxamine (*Desferal*) chelates iron.
      a. It must be administered **parenterally.**
      b. Hemochromatosis is an indication for use.

4. Edetate calcium disodium **(EDTA)** (*Calcium Disodium Versenate*) binds many heavy metals, but is used primarily to treat lead poisoning.

   a. It must be administered **parenterally.**

   b. **Nephrotoxicity** is a major limitation of this chelator.

B. Heavy metals form chelates with natural substances in the body. It is this phenomenon which leads to their toxicity.

   1. **Lead** is handled much like calcium in the body.

   a. **Accumulation** occurs first **in soft tissues** (e.g., kidney), and then **in bone, teeth, and hair.**

   b. Lead can be mobilized from bone by parathyroid hormone.

   c. **Chronic poisoning** from lead is the most common problem, and the symptoms are diverse and non-specific, including:

   (1) **Neurologic effects** (e.g., mental retardation, especially in children)

   (2) **GI lead colic**

   (3) **Peripheral neuritis**

   (4) **Nephropathy**

   (5) **Anemias**

   d. **Treatment** involves the use of chelators.

   (1) Both **calcium disodium EDTA** and **dimercaprol** are used initially.

   (2) **Sodium EDTA is not used** because it will chelate endogenous calcium and can induce hypocalcemic tetany.

   (3) Long-term deleading is performed with **oral penicillamine** or oral succimer (*Chemet*), another lead chelator.

   2. **Mercury** forms covalent bonds with sulphur-containing compounds.

   a. **Cell membranes and enzymes** (e.g., cytochrome oxidase) are damaged.

   b. **Acute poisoning** can occur by several routes of exposure.

   (1) Ingestion of mercury induces a **GI syndrome.**

   (2) Inhalation induces a **pneumonitis.**

   (3) **Renal tubular necrosis** occurs with any route of exposure.

   c. **Chronic poisoning** leads to:

   (1) **Neurologic complications,** especially with methylmercury, which is very lipid-soluble.

   (2) **Nephrotoxicity**

   d. **Treatment** of acute mercury poisoning involves the administration of:

   (1) **Fluids**

   (2) **Chelators**

   (a) **Dimercaprol** is used for mercury salt poisoning.

   (b) **Penicillamine** is used for mercury vapor poisoning.

   (c) None are effective for methylmercury poisoning.

   3. **Arsenic** binds sulfhydryl groupings which leads to enzyme inhibition, or substitutes for phosphate in adenosine triphosphate (ATP).

   a. **Acute** poisoning induces:

   (1) **GI syndromes**

   (2) **Circulatory collapse**

   b. **Chronic** arsenic poisoning leads to **peripheral neuropathies.**

   c. A diagnostic feature is a **garlic odor** on the breath.

   d. **Treatment** of acute arsenic poisoning involves the administration of:

   (1) **Fluids**

   (2) **Vasopressors**

   (3) **Dimercaprol**

    e. Treatment of chronic arsenic poisoning involves the administration of **dimercaprol or penicillamine.**

  4. Iron is very corrosive to the GI tract if taken in high dosages.
    a. Acute ingestion induces a **hemorrhagic GI necrosis,** resulting in the development of **shock and metabolic acidosis.**
    b. Treatment involves:
      (1) **Lavage with bicarbonate,** which yields ferrous carbonate, a substance that is not absorbed
      (2) Fluids
      (3) Correction of the acidosis
      (4) Deferoxamine

III. OTHER TOXIC SUBSTANCES

  A. Carbon monoxide induces hypoxia.

    1. It acts by:
      a. **Forming carboxyhemoglobin.** The affinity of carbon monoxide for hemoglobin is 200 times greater than the affinity of oxygen for hemoglobin.
      b. **Decreasing the dissociation of oxygen** from oxyhemoglobin.

    2. Treatment for carbon monoxide toxicity involves one of the following:
      a. Inhalation of fresh air
      b. Artificial ventilation
      c. 100% oxygen, which shortens the half-life of the carboxyhemoglobin

  B. Cyanide has a high affinity for ferric (Fe^{3+}) iron.

    1. **Cytochrome oxidases** in mitochondria, which contain Fe^{3+}, are inhibited.
      a. Cellular respiration is decreased.
      b. A cytotoxic hypoxia is induced.

    2. The specific **treatment** for poisoning includes administration of:
      a. A nitrite to induce **methemoglobinemia;** which binds cyanide, drawing it off the cytochrome oxidases
      b. **Thiosulfate,** which converts the cyanide on the methemoglobin to thiocyanate which is excreted

  C. Hydrogen sulfide also **inhibits cytochrome oxidases. Treatment** involves the administration of **nitrites** to induce **methemoglobinemia,** which binds the sulfide.

  D. Carbon tetrachloride (a halogenated hydrocarbon) has many toxic effects.

    1. Acute poisoning leads to:
      a. **CNS depression** with respiratory depression
      b. **Arrhythmias,** due to the sensitization of the myocardium to catecholamines

    2. Chronic poisoning leads to a disruption of cell membranes, resulting in:
      a. Hepatotoxicity
      b. Nephrotoxicity

  E. Dichlorodiphenyltrichloroethane **(DDT) is very lipid soluble.**

    1. It is **concentrated in fat.**
      a. Elimination from the body is extremely slow (1% / day).
      b. It gets into the **food chain,** and biomagnification occurs.

    2. Acute toxicity results from the **blockade of potassium permeability changes in**

nerve membranes. This can induce tremors and convulsions, although death does not occur in humans.

F. **Paraquat** increases the formation of a **superoxide anion radical** which attacks lipids and produces **pulmonary injury.**

G. **Thalidomide** is a teratogen which **alters organogenesis** (the action of most teratogens), leading to **phocomelia.**